BREAST CANCER

An Annotated Guide to the Current Literature

BREAST CANCER

An Annotated Guide to the Current Literature

Edited by

N. G. Arashvili

NOVA SCIENCE PUBLISHERS, INC.

Art Director: Christopher Concannon
Graphics: Elenor Kallberg and Maria Ester Hawrys
Manuscript Coordinator: Roseann Pena
Book Production: Tammy Sauter, Benjamin Fung
and Michelle Lalo
Circulation: Irene Kwartiroff and Annette Hellinger

Library of Congress Cataloging–in–Publication Data
available upon request

ISBN 1-56072-112-X

6080 Jericho Turnpike, Suite 207
Commack, New York 11725
Tele. 516-499-3103 Fax 516-499-3146
E Mail Novasci1@aol.com

Printed in the United States of America

BREAST CANCER

An Annotated Guide to the Current Literature

CONTENTS

NOVA SCIENCE PUBLISHERS, INC.

BC0001 BREAST CANCER: NEW KEYS TO EARLY DETECTION

McCall's

Mar. 1987, vol. 114, p. 83 (2)
Detection
How to do breast self-examination. Types of cancer women get.

BC0002 THINKING ABOUT BREAST CANCER

U.S. News and World Report

May 18, 1987, vol. 102, p. 65(1)
Women

BC0003 SCREENING FOR CERVICAL AND BREAST CANCER-SOUTHEASTERN KENTUCKY

JAMA: The Journal of the American Medical Association

Feb. 26, 1988, vol. 259, n. n8, p. 1141(2)
Kentucky

BC0004 TREATMENT FOR VERY EARLY CANCER

Consumer Reports

Nov. 1988, vol. 53, n. n11, p. 733(1)
Early cancer

BC0005 SCREENING RECOMMENDATIONS FOR THE ELDERLY

American Journal of Public Elderly

Sept. 1991, vol. 81, p. 1131-1140
Medical Care

BC0006 BREAST CANCER PREDICTION AND THE WOLFE CLASSIFICATION OF MAMMOGRAMS

Journal of the American Medical Association

Aug. 23-30, 1985, vol. 254, p. 1050-1053
Medical Screening

BC0007 BREAST CANCER SCREENING AMONG RELATIVES OF WOMEN WITH BREAST CANCER

American Journal of Public Health

Sept. 1991, vol. 81, p. 1174-1179
Health surveys; medical statistics

BC0008 CANCER SCREENING INTERVENTION AMONG BLACK WOMEN IN INNER-CITY ATLANTA--DESIGN OF A STUDY

Public Health Report

July-Aug. 1992, vol. 107, p. 381-388
Atlanta, Black Women

BC0009 MAMMOGRAPHIC SCREENING IN ASYMPTOMATIC WOMEN AGED 40 YEARS AND OLDER

Journal of the American Medical Association

May 5, 1989, vol. 261, p. 2535-2542
Women's health services

BC0010 THE DEBATE OVER THE MASS MAMMOGRAPHY IN BRITAIN

British Medical Journal

Oct. 15, 1988, vol. 297, p. 969-972
Britian; Mammography

BC0011 DOES INCREASED DETECTION ACCOUNT FOR THE RISING INCIDENCE OF BREAST CANCER?

American Journal of Public Health

Apr. 1991, vol. 81, p. 461-465
Detection

BC0012 INCREASING THE EFFORT TOWARD BREAST CANCER DETECTION

Journal of the American Medical Association

Mar. 14, 1986, vol. 255, p. 1311-1315
Detection

BC0013 MULTISTRATEGY HEALTH EDUCATION PROGRAM TO INCREASE MAMMOGRAPHY USE AMONG WOMEN AGES 65 AND OLDER

Public Health Report

July-Aug. 1992, vol. 107, p. 369-380
Medical Screening; medical care

BC0014 CANCER DETECTION IN WOMEN

Washington G.P.O.

Jan. 28, 1988, p. 250
Women's health services, Detection

BC0015 THE VALUE OF MAMMOGRAPHY SCREENING IN WOMEN UNDER AGE 50 YEARS

Journal of the American Medical Association

Mar. 11, 1988, vol. 259, p. 1512-1519
Risk assessment; imaging systems in medicine

BC0016 EARLY BREAST CANCER: HISTOPATHOLOGY, DIAGNOSIS, AND TREATMENT

1985, P. 321
Early cancer; Histopathology

BC0017 INTERNATIONAL WORKSHOP ON MONOCLONAL ANTIBODIES AND BREAST CANCER

1985, p. 314
Diagnosis

BC0018 TUMOR MARKERS AND THEIR SIGNIFICANCE IN THE MANAGEMENT OF BREAST CANCER: PROCEEDINGS OF A WORKSHOP HELD IN BETHESDA

1986, p. 147
Diagnosis

BC0019 BREAST CANCER: DIAGNOSIS AND TREATMENT

1987, vol. XIII, p. 577
Diagnosis

BC0020 BREAST CANCER: PRESENT PERSPECTIVE OF EARLY DIAGNOSIS

Third International Copenhagen Symposium on Detection of Breast

1987, vol. VIII, p. 132
Diagnosis

BC0021 BREAST CANCER DETECTION: THE NEED FOR A FEDERAL RESPONSE

Subcommittee on Health and Long-Term Care

1986, p. 169
Radiography

BC0022 DIAGNOSTIC HISTOPATHOLOGY OF THE BREAST

1987, p. 362
Cytodiagnosis

BC0023 BREAST CANCER DETECTION: MAMMOGRAPHY AND OTHER METHODS IN BREAST IMAGING

1987, vol. XVI, p. 204
Mammography

BC0024 DIAGNOSIS AND MANAGEMENT OF BREAST CANCER

1988, vol. XI, p. 569

BC0025 IMMUNOLOGICAL APPROACHES TO THE DIAGNOSIS AND THERAPY OF BREAST CANCER

International Workshop on Monoclonal antibodies and Breast

1987, vol. X, p. 272
Immunogical Therapy

BC0026 SCREENING FOR BREAST CANCER

1988, vol. VIII, p. 124
Screening

BC0027 BREAST SCREENING: REPORT TO THE HEALTH MINISTERS OF ENGLAND, WALES, SCOTLAND AND NORTHERN IRELAND

1986, p. 102
England, Wales, Scotland

BC0028 CONTROVERSIES IN BREAST DISEASE: DIAGNOSIS AND MANAGEMENT

1988, vol. XV, p. 514

BC0029 CANCER DETECTION IN WOMEN

Committee on Labor and Human Resources

Jan. 28, 1988, vol. III, p. 250
Detection

BC0030 HIGH-RISK BREAST CANCER: DIAGNOSIS

1989, vol. IX, p. 383

BC0031 BREAST CANCER IMMUNODIAGNOSIS AND IMMUNOTHERAPY

Proceedings of the Third International Workshop on Monoclonal

1989, vol. XI, p. 259
Immunodiagsis; Immunotherapy

BC0032 PRACTICAL MODALITIES OF AN EFFICIENT SCREENING FOR BREAST CANCER IN THE EUROPEAN COMMUNITY

Proceedings of an International Symposium of the Association

1989, vol. XIII, p. 211
Europe; Screening

BC0033 MAKE SURE YOU DO NOT HAVE BREAST CANCER

1989, vol. XXIV, p. 118
Strax, Philip

BC0034 INFORMATION SYSTEMS IN BREAST CANCER DETECTION

International Workshop on Information Systems in Breast Cancer

1990
Detection

BC0035 FILM-SCREEN MAMMOGRAPHY: AN ATLAS OF INSTRUCTIONAL CASES

1991, p. 312
Mammography

BC0036 ADVANCES IN BREAST CANCER DETECTION

Fourth International Copenhagen Symposium on Detection of Breast

1990, vol. IX, p. 195
Detection

BC0037 TREATMENT OF PRECANCEROUS LESIONS AND EARLY BREAST CANCER

1993
Early cancer; Precancer

BC0038 TEXTBOOK OF MAMMOGRAPHY

1993
Radiography

BC0039 BREAST CANCER: MAMMOGRAPHY AND BREAST EXAMINATION ARE THE BEST METHODS FOR EARLY DETECTION

Mayo Clinic Health Letter

Apr. 1990, vol. 8, n. n4, p. 6(2)
Mammography

BC0040 SCREENING MAMMOGRAPHY: A MISSED CLINICAL OPPORTUNITY

The Journal of the American Medical Association

July 4, 1990, vol. 264, n. n1, p. 54(5)
Mammography

Research studies have clearly shown that mortality from breast cancer can be reduced by regular breast cancer screening for early detection, yet this preventive health measure is still underutilized in the United States. The National Cancer Institute (NCI) has set a goal for at least 80 percent of all women aged 50 to 70 to have an annual breast examination and mammogram by the year 2000. To reach this goal, the NCI sponsored seven studies in different communities to determine how many women are currently having breast cancer screening, and for those who are not, why they are not. The women surveyed in all the studies were aged 50 to 74 and did not have breast cancer. The number of women in each study ranged from 277 to 2,180 and all were non-hispanic whites. It was found that over 90 percent of the women had a regular physician, but not all of them had either a clinical breast examination (in which the breast are examined for lumps by a health professional) or a mammogram, an X-ray of the breast. In the past year, more women (46 to 76 percent) had a clinical breast exam than had a mammogram (25 to 41 percent). Women who had a low income or less education had fewer mammograms. When women were asked why they had not had a mammogram, the two most common reasons were that they did not know they needed to, and that their doctor had not suggested it. The author conclude that a large number of physicians are missing the opportunity to recommend mammograms for their older women patients. (Consumer Summary produced by Reliance Medical Information, Inc.) Characteristics of study populations. (table) Breast cancer screening rates. (graph) Percentage of white women who had a mammogram in past year. (table) Percentage of white women who had a clinical breast exam. (table) Reasons women gave for never having had a mammogram. (table)

BC0041 MAMMOGRAPHY SCREENING: IS IT SAFE?

Ms.

Sept.-Oct. 1990, vol. 1, n. n2, p. 31(1)
Mammography

BC0042 MEDICARE EXTENDS COVERAGE FOR PAP SMEARS, ADDS MAMMOGRAMS

Aging Winter

1991, n. n362, p. 42(2)
Medical screening; Cervical cancer

BC0043 MAMMOGRAPHY: DON'T NEGLECT THIS LIFESAVING TEST

Good Housekeeping

Feb. 1991, vol. 212, n. n2, p. 127(2)
Pap test

BC0044 MAMMOGRAPHY SCREENING ADDED TO BUDGET PACKAGE
Modern Maturity
Feb.-Mar. 1991, vol. 34, n. n1, p. 9(1)
Mammography

BC0045 BREAST SELF-EXAMINATION IN RELATION TO THE OCCURRENCE OF ADVANCED BREAST CANCER
The Journal of the American Medical Association
May, 8, 1991, vol. 265, n. n18, p. 2331(1)
Self Examination

BC0046 SHARPER IMAGING FOR BREASTS
Glamour
Apr. 1992, vol. 90, n. n4, p. 45(1)
Imaging

BC0047 BREAST-CANCER ADVANCES
Consumers Digest
May-June 1992, vol. 31, n. n3, p. 84(2)

BC0048 ARE MAMMOGRAMS BAD FOR YOUR HEALTH?
Time
May 18, 1992, vol. 139, n. n20, p. 25(1)
Mammograms

BC0049 PUBLIC HEALTH FOCUS: MAMMOGRAPHY
The Journal of the American Medical Association
July 22, 1992, vol. 268, n. n452(2)
Mammography
The number of newly-diagnosed cases of breast cancer increase between 1980 and 1987, but the death rate remained stable. This may be a result of mammography, which can detect tumors before they become large enough to bet detected by breast examination. Screening women at risk for breast cancer may be one way to reduce mortality. In fact, studies have shown that mammographic screening can reduce mortality as much as 39 percent in women over 50 years old. The benefit of mammographic screening in younger women has yet to be documented. Estimates of the cost-effectiveness of mammography in women over 50 vary, from $4,500 for each year of life saved to over $84,000. Mammography could be cost effective if more sensitive film is used and more women participate regularly. It is also important to develop a mechanism to refer women with an abnormal mammogram to the appropriate treatment program.

BC0050 BREAST CANCER: ORIGINS, DETECTION, AND TREATMENT
Proceedings of the International Breast Cancer Research Conference
1986, vol. XVII, p. 343
Detection

BC0051 DIAGNOSTIC BREAST PATHOLOGY: A COLOUR ATLAS AND TEXT
Ahmed, Ali
1992
Pathology

BC0052 MAMMOGRAPHY TRIAL COMES UNDER FIRE
Allison, M.; M.
Science
May 22, 1992, vol. 256, n. n5060, p. 1128(3)
Mammography

BC0053 BREAST CANCER SCREENING
Austoker, J.
1988, vol. VIII, p. 54
Screening

BC0054 BREAST CANCER SCREENING
Austoker, J.
1989
Screening

BC0055 WHO FEARS BREAST EXAMS?
Baker, S.
Health
Feb. 1991, vol. 23, n. n1, p. 17(1)
Fear

BC0056 ATLAS OF BREAST DISEASE
Barth, V.
1991, vol. IX, p. 262

BC0057 DIFFERENCES IN RATES OF CANCER SCREENING BY USUAL SOURCE OF MEDICAL CARE
Bernstein, A.B.;
Medical Care
Mar. 1991, vol. 29, p. 196-209
Health maintenance organizations

BC0058 BREAST CANCER
Bowe, C.; D. Birk
Cosmopolitan
Feb. 1991, vol. 210, n. n2, p. 148(4)

BC0059 ONE WOMAN'S BATTLE AGAINST CANCER
Brooks, H. and R.
50 Plus
June 1986, vol. 26, p. 34(5)
Mastectomy
Jeanne Rogers

BC0060 THE ACCEPTANCE AND COMPLETION OF MAMMOGRAPHY BY OLDER BLACK WOMEN
Burack, R.C. and
American Journal of Public Health
June 1989, vol. 79, p. 721-726
Black Women; Mammography

BC0061 AUTHORITIES BACK MAMMOGRAPHY SCREENING
Buterbaugh, L.
Medical World News
June 1992, vol. 33, n. n6, p. 25(2)
Black Women; Mammography
Health authorities do not agree with a Canadian study that indicates that mammograms do not lead to decreased mortality. The American Cancer Society continues to encourage women to have mammograms before they reach the age of 50.

BC0062 INTERPRETATION OF BREAST BIOPSIES
Carter, D.
1990, vol. X, p. 246
Biopsies

BC0063 DOCTORS AREN'T DETECTING CANCER IN TIME

Castelman, M.
Redbook
Oct. 1986, vol. 167, p. 138(4)
Colorectal cancer; Detecting

BC0064 BREASTS: YOUR PERSONAL GUIDE

Chatman, W.
Teen
July 1991, vol. 35, n. n7, p. 86(3)
Self-examination, Medical

BC0065 BREAST CANCER TREATMENTS

Cimons, M.; A.
50 Plus
Oct. 1990, vol. 30, n. n10, p. 44(3)
Lumpectomy; Mastectomy; Mammography

BC0066 PREDICTION OF RELAPSE OR SURVIVAL IN PATIENTS WITH NODE-NEGATIVE BREAST CANCER DY DNA FLOW CYTOMETRY

Clark, G.M.; L.G.
The New England Journal of Medicine
Mar. 9, 1989, vol. 320, n. n10, p. 627(7)
DNA Flow Cytometry

BC0067 PREDICTION OF RELAPSE OR SURVIVAL IN PATIENTS WITH NODE-NEGATIVE BREAST CANCER BY DNA FLOW CYTOMETRY

Clark, G.M.; L.G.
The New England Journal of Medicine
Mar. 9, 1989, vol. 320, n. n10, p. 627(7)
DNA Flow Cytometry; Relapse

In approximately half of the women diagnosed with breast cancer, the disease is restricted to the breast itself, with no evidence of cancer cells found in the neighboring lymph nodes. The availability of early breast cancer detection has made the diagnosis of more node-negative cancers. Even though the prognosis is good, 30 percent of the women with no modal involvement die from the cancer. Treatment of node-negative breast cancers is controversial, and some practitioners give extra therapy. Factors influencing prognosis may help physicians select those patients who would benefit the most from such potentially toxic additional therapy. Most from such potentially toxic additional therapy. Diseased tissue in 395 frozen samples was analyzed for specific cell type and behavior by DNA flow-cytometry. Patients with aneuploid (cells with abnormal amount of chromosomes) tumors had five-year survival rates of 74 percent, compared with 88 percent among patients with diploid tumors (normal number of chromosomes). In the latter case, low S-phase fractions (a specific synthesis phase of a cell cycle) indicated 90 percent survival at five years and high values indicated a survival of 70 percent. This method of evaluating the characteristics of tumor cells is a meaningful indicator of survival of node-negative breast cancer patients. Patients with diploid, low S-phase tumors have good prognosis and may not be good candidates for adjuvant therapy. Tumor specimen characteristics that could be evaluated for ploidy status. (table) Multivariate survival analyses in all patients (N=345). (table) Disease-free survival according to ploidy status. (graph) Multivariate survival analyses in patients with diploid tumors (N=112). (table) Disease-free and overall survival rates at 5 years according to aneuploidy. (table) Disease-free survival according to prognostic group. (graph)

BC0068 A NEEDLE INSTEAD OF A KNIFE
Cowley, G.
Newsweek
Apr. 13, 1992, vol. 119, n. n15, p. 62(1)
Diagnosis; Biopsy

BC0069 UNRELIABLE BREAST CANCER SCREENING HALTED
Cramer, T.; R. Mishra
FDA Consumer
Nov. 1991, vol. 25, n. n9, p. 42(2)
Diagnostic equipment industry; Transillumination

BC0070 AFFIRMATIONS, MEDITATIONS, AND ENCOURAGEMENTS FOR WOMEN LIVING WITH BREAST CANCER
Dackman, L.
1991
Women

BC0071 AFFIRMATIONS, MEDITATIONS, AND ENCOURAGEMENTS FOR WOMEN LIVING WITH BREAST CANCER
Dackman, L.
1993
Women

BC0072 BIOPSY OF OCCULT BREAST LESIONS AND PROFESSIONAL LIABILITY
Darios, R.J.; M.R. J.E. Meyer;
The Journal of the American Medical Association
Oct. 17, 1990, vol. 264, n. n15, p. 1948(1)
Mammography; Biopsies

BC0073 ATLAS OF FILM-SCREEN MAMMOGRAPHY
De Paredes, E.S.
1989, p. 364
Mammography

BC0074 ATLAS OF FILM-SCREEN MAMMOGRAPHY
De Paredes, E.S.
1992, p. 628
Mammography

BC0075 CANCER AND BREAST LUMPS
Edmonson, D.
Parents
Sept. 1985, vol. 60, p. 16(1)
Lumps

BC0076 THE INFLUENCE OF DIAGNOSTIC RADIOGRAPHY ON THE INCIDENCE OF BREAST CANCER AND LEUKEMIA
Evans, J.S.; J.E.
The New England Journal of Medicine
Sept. 25, 1986, vol. 315, p. 810-815
X-rays; Health surveys

BC0077 PREDICTING THE RETURN OF BREAST CANCER
Fackelmann, K.A.
Science News
Apr. 11, 1992, vol. 141, n. n15, p. 239(1)
Obesity

BC0078 THE DETECTION AND TREATMENT OF EARLY BREAST CANCER

Fentiman, I.S.

1990, p. 272
Early Cancer

BC0079 PHYSICIANS' ABILITIES TO DETECT LUMPS IN SILICONE BREAST MODELS

Fletcher, S.W.;

Journal of the American Medical Association

Apr. 19, 1985, vol. 253, p. 2224-2228
Lumps

BC0080 THE WAR ON BREAST CANCER

Foreman, J.

Ladies' Home Journal

Oct. 1988, vol. 105, n. n10, p. 141(8)
The stages of breast cancer.

BC0081 THE EFFECT OF PHYSICIAN-PATIENT COMMUNICATION ON MAMMOGRAPHY UTILIZATION BY DIFFERENT ETHNIC GROUPS

Fox, S.A. and J.A.

Medical Care

Nov. 1991, vol. 29, p. 1065-1082
Mammography

BC0082 BREAST SELF-EXAMINATION IN YOUNG WOMEN: MORE HARM THAN GOOD?

Frank, J.W. and V.

Lancet

Sept. 21, 1985, no. 8456, p. 654-657
Health surveys, Self Examination

BC0083 GETTING AN EXPERT MAMMOGRAM

Gertz, K.R.

Town and Country

Nov. 1991, vol. 145, n. n5138, p. 170(7)
Mammogram

BC0084 EARLY DETECTION, EARLY CURE

Gutfeld, G.; M.

Prevention

May 1992, vol. 44, n. n5, p. 22(2)
Early Cancer

BC0085 HOSPITAL VARIABLES ASSOCIATED WITH QUALITY OF CARE FOR BREAST CANCER PATIENTS

Hand, R.; S. Sener;
The Journal of the American Medical Association
Dec. 25, 1991, vol. 266, n. n24, p. 3429(4)
Hospital

The prognosis for patients with breast cancer is improved with early detection and proper treatment of the disease. Screening mammography (breast X-ray) is widely used to detect breast cancer in its early stages. Certain treatments are recommended for specific findings. This study examined the attributes of hospitals that contributed to quality care for breast cancer patients. quality of care was defined by a hospital's use of five variables that contribute to better patient outcome. These variables include: early detection, hormone receptor determination, adjuvant therapy when indicated, radiation therapy when indicated, and ancillary lymph node dissection when indicated. Although over 90 percent of all cases were detected early, at some hospitals more than 23 percent of breast cancer patients were diagnosed in late stages. Attributed associated with such hospitals included an urban location, many poorly insured patients, and fewer breast cancer patients treated. Failure of hospitals to use two of the variables, adjuvant therapy and radiation therapy, was widely reported with wide ranges between hospitals. No hospital attributes were shown to be related t omission of adjuvant therapy. Omission of radiation therapy was associated with urban location and few breast cancer patients. These results indicate that treatment of breast cancer is less than optimal at many small, urban hospitals that are poorly funded. (Consumer Summary produced by Reliance Medical Information. Inc.) Hospital variables. (table) Stage distribution of breast cancer patients. (table) quality variables calculated for each hospital. (table) Proportion of variance of quality variables. (table)

BC0086 NONPALPABLE BREAST CANCER: DIAGNOSIS AND MANAGEMENT

Hermann, G.
1992, vol. X, p. 132
Nonpalpable Cancer

BC0087 MEDICAL BREAKTHROUGHS YOU MUST KNOW ABOUT

Hochman, G.
Ladies' Home Journal
Mar. 1988, vol. 105, n. n3, p. 90(3)
Ampligen(medication; L-deprenyl; enalapril; AIDS-related complex; Alzheimer's disease; arthritis; methotrexate; azathioprine; heart

BC0088 INTERACTIVE VIDEO PROMOTES PATIENT-DOCTOR PARTNERSHIP

Holzman, D.
Business and Health
Mar. 1992, vol. 10, p. 42, 46-49
Interactive Video

BC0089 MAMMOGRAM ALERT

Hunt, D.
East West
Sept.-Oct. 1991, vol. 21, p. 55-59, 108-109
X-rays

BC0090 CATCHING A KILLER; EARLY DETECTION CAN DECREASE CASES OF BREAST CANCER

Keating, J. Jr.
New Orleans
Apr. 1985, vol. 19, p. 54(1)
Detection

BC0091 NOT EVERYONE AGREES WITH NEW MAMMOGRAPHIC SCREENING GUIDELINES DESIGNED TO END CONFUSION

King, A.S.
The Journal of the American Medical Association
Sept. 1, 1989, vol. 262, n. n9, p. 1154(2)
Medical care, cost of

Mammographic screening guidelines suggested by the National Medical Roundtable have provoked debate. Breast cancer is the most common cancer among U.S. women accounts for more than 28 percent of malignant tumors. Estimates for 1989 project that more than 142,000 new cases of breast cancer will be diagnosed and 43,000 women will die as a result of the disease. One of the best means of lowering these mortality rates is early detection: when breast cancer is detected before it has spread five-year survival rates exceed 85 percent. Many experts feel that mammography, X-ray examination of the breast, is the best means of detecting the cancer during its most curable stage. Although the value of mammography for women aged 40 to 49 years who may be at risk for breast cancer is not in dispute, controversy was caused by the new recommendation that all women in this age range undergo mammography every one to two years. Women in this age group account for less than 10 percent of all breast cancers. Critics argue that there is lack of conclusive evidence demonstrating the benefits of breast cancer screening for women aged 40 to 49 who are not at risk and have no symptoms of breast cancer and that the cost of mass screening would outweigh its benefits. Insurance often does not cover the cost of screening mammography although some states are passing laws requiring insurance companies to pay for these procedures. The cost of screening mammography is being reduced from $125 to $50 as more centers capable of providing low-cost mammographic exams are established. The controversy over breast cancer screening will continue until more is learned about the causes of the disease and the use of mammography in early detection.

BC0092 BREAST

Kline, T.S.
1989, vol. XIII, p. 253

BC0093 BREAST CANCER: ANGUISH, MYSTERY AND HOPE

Kolata, G.
New York Times Magazine
Apr. 24, 1988, p. 43,70,73, 96-97
Cancer research; National Cancer Institute

BC0094 MAMMOGRAM ALERT: WHAT CAN GO RIGHT, WHAT CAN GO WRONG

Kolata, G.
Redbook
Aug. 1991, vol. 177, n. n4, p. 58(3)
Mammograms

BC0095 BREAST IMAGING

Kopans, D.B.
1989, vol. XIII, p. 375
Imaging

BC0096 BREAST CANCER: UNRAVELING THE CONFUSING REPORTS
Lake, A. and G.
Woman's Day
Apr. 18, 1989, p. 84(4)

BC0097 BREAST CANCER SCREENING PRACTICES AMONG USERS OF COUNTY-FUNDED HEALTH CENTERS VS WOMEN IN THE ENTIRE COMMUNITY
Lane, D.S.; A.P.
American Journal of Public Health
Feb. 1992, vol. 82, p. 199-203
Women's health services; Health surveys

BC0098 ONCOGENES AND BREAST CANCER
Lippman, M.E.
The New England Journal of Medicine
Nov. 10, 1988, vol. 319, n. n19, p. 1281(2)
Antineoplastic agents

BC0099 BREAST CANCER: EARLY DECISIONS
Love, S.
The Harvard Medical School Health Letter
Mar. 1988, vol. 13, n. n5, p. 1(4)
Intraductal carcinoma in situ
Breast cross-section.

BC0100 SOFTWARE THAT SPOTS BREAST CANCER EARLY
Marbach, W.D.
Business Week
July 27, 1992, n. n3276, p. 83(1)
Mammography

BC0101 PROGRESS IN PREDICTING BREAST CANCER RELAPSES
Marx, J.L.
Science
July 29, 1988, vol. 241, n. n4865, p. 535(1)
Genetic screening; oncogenes

BC0102 A NEW VIEW OF BREAST CANCER
McCabe, C.
American Health
July-Aug. 1992, vol. 11, n. n6, p. 14(1)
Magnetic resonance imaging

BC0103 THE TENDER BUD: A PHYSICIAN'S JOURNEY THROUGH BREAST CANCER
Meldin, M.
1992

BC0104 BREAST DEFENSE
Morici, J.
Weight Watchers
Nov. 1988, vol. 21, n. n10, p. 16(2)
Breast cancer detection methods.

BC0105 BREAST-CANCER RESEARCHERS TRY NEW TECHNIQUE
Nazario, S.L.
The Wall Street Journal
July 31, 1992, p. B1(W) pB1

BC0106 SCREENING FOR BREAST CANCER WITH BREAST SELF-EXAMINATION; A CRITICAL REVIEW

O'Malley, M. S.
JAMA: The Journal of the American Medical Association
Apr. 24, 1987, vol. 257, p. 2197(7)
Self-examination

Criteria for determining the appropriateness of screening. Descriptive studies of the effectiveness of treatment. Estimated sensitivity for breast examination.

BC0107 SCREENING FOR BREAST CANCER WITH SELF-EXAMINATION: A CRITICAL REVIEW

O'Malley, M.S.
Journal of the American Medical Association
Apr. 24, 1987, vol. 257, p. 2197-2203
Screening

BC0108 FINE NEEDLE ASPIRATION OF THE BREAST

Oertel, Y.C.
1987, vol. XIV, p. 203
Fine Needle Aspiration

BC0109 THE CASE OF THE SUSPECT LUMP

Padus, E.
Prevention
Aug. 1989, vol. 41, n. n8, p. 112(5)
Lumps

BC0110 PROLIFERATIVE BREAST DISEASE: DIAGNOSIS AND IMPLICATIONS

Page, D.L.; W.D.
Science
Aug. 26, 1991, vol. 111, n. n9, p. 68(2)
Proliferative Breast Cancer

BC0111 IMMUNOCYTOCHEMISTRY FOR STEROID RECEPTORS

Pertschuk, L.P.
1990, p. 210
Immunodiagnosis

BC0112 HIGH-TECH CANCER TESTS

Polevoy, M.
American Health
Sept. 1992, vol. 11, n. n7, p. 9(3)
Prostate cancer; Ovarian cancer; Bladder cancer; Colorectal cancer; Lung Cancer

BC0113 ANTIBODIES PINPOINT MIGRATING MINI-TUMORS

Raloff, J.
Science News
June 1, 1991, vol. 139, n. n22, p. 340(1)
Antibodies

BC0114 BREAST CANCER THERAPY'S LEUKEMIA RISKS

Raloff, J.
Science News
June 27, 1992, vol. 141, n. n26, p. 420(1)
Leukemic

BC0115 MULTISTRATEGY HEALTH EDUCATION PROGRAM TO INCREASE MAMMOGRAPHY USE AMONG WOMEN AGES 65 AND OLDER

Rimer, B.K.; N.
Public Health Reports
July-Aug. 1992, vol. 107, n. n4, p. 369(12)

BC0116 NEW SCREENING MAY REPLACE BREAST BIOPSY

Ruiz, A.T.
McCall's
May 1991, vol. 118, n. n8, p. 30(1)
Screening

BC0117 THE SEVERITY OF BREAST CANCER AT DIAGNOSIS: A COMPARISON OF AGE AND EXTENT OF DISEASE IN BLACK AND WHITE WOMEN

Satariano, W.A.;
American Journal of Public Health
July 1986, vol. 76, p. 779-782
Black

BC0118 A MINIMALIST POLICY FOR BREAST CANCER SURVEILLANCE

Schapira, D.V.
The Journal of the American Medical Association
Jan. 16, 1991, vol. 265, n. n3, p. 380(3)

Breast cancer patients (stage I or II cancer) are usually followed-up to detect tumor recurrence, with the idea that such surveillance improves survival. Surveillance programs usually include a physical examination (with mammogram) and blood tests, including measurement of factors known to be associated with malignancy. Evidence exists, however, that shows such surveillance does not improve survival. This evidence is reviewed and evaluated. At least three quarters of all cases of breast cancer recurrence are discovered by patients themselves between follow-up visits; in one study, physicians found abnormalities in only 15 percent of the cases. Bone scans to detect metastases (cancer spread) have a high rate of false-positive results; only one in nine patients with abnormal results actually have bone metastases. Chest X-rays were not useful in detecting recurrence: one study showed that recurrence was detected by this method in only 2 percent of patients. Finally, evaluation of blood chemistry to diagnose liver function rarely show recurrence in patients who did not already have symptoms of metastasis, and some test results were elevated in women without metastasis.

BC0119 DUCTAL CARCINOMA IN SITU

Schnitt, S. J.; W.
The New England Journal of Medicine
Apr. 7, 1988, vol. 318, n. n14, 898(6)
Ductal Carcinoma

Results of treatment of ductal carcinoma in situ.

BC0120 A 42-YEAR-OLD WOMAN WITH DYSPONEA AND DIFFUSE INTERSTITIAL PULMONARY DISEASE

Scully, R.E. Mark, E.J. McNeely, McNeely,
The New England Journal of Medicine
Aug. 2, 1990, vol. 323, n. n5, p. 327(8)
Shortness of breath; Respiratory distress syndrome; Pneumonia

BC0121 BREAST CANCER: COMPLACENCY THE ENEMY OF CURE

Segal, M.
FDA Consumer
July-Aug. 1991, vol. 25, n. n6, p. 7(7)
Cures
About half of all breast cancers develop in the upper outer quadrant. (chart) Anatomy of the breast. (chart)

BC0122 ACUTE, DIFFUSE, NONTENDER EDEMA OF THE LEFT BREAST IN A 50-YEAR-OLD WOMAN

Seibel, D.G.; K.D.
JAMA: The Journal of the American Medical Association
Sept. 18, 1987, vol. 258, p. 1515(2)
Edema

BC0123 MEDICAL MAILBOX

Servaas, C.
The Saturday Evening Post
July-Aug. 1986, vol. 258, p. 106(3)
Mammography; Medical screening; Diagnostic services

BC0124 THE MAMMOBILE GOES TO WASHINGTON

Servaas, C.
The Saturday Evening Post
Oct. 1986, vol. 258, p. 50(8)
Diet
Size of breast cancers detected by various means.

BC0125 PROSTATE MANOGRAMS ON THE MALEMOBILE

Servaas, C.
The Saturday Evening Post
Jan.-Feb. 1987, vol. 259, p. 106(4)
Prostate cancer; rectum; insulin; diabetes

BC0126 PREVENT BREAST CANCER DEATHS

SerVaas, C.
Saturday Evening Post
Mar. 1986, vol. 258, p. 68-71
X-rays

BC0127 HOW TO BEAT BREAST CANCER

Silberner, J.
U.S. News and World Report
July 11, 1988, vol. 105, n. n2, p. 52(9)
Mammography
Breast cancers per 100,000 women. Share of all women surveyed who have had a mammogram. Reasons cited for having a mammogram during the last two years. The five stages of breast cancer. Where to go for help and hope.

BC0128 FALSE PREMISES AND FALSE PROMISES OF BREAST CANCER SCREENING

Skrabanek, P.
Lancet
Aug. 10, 1985, no. 8450, p. 316-320
Screening

BC0129 INCREASING PHYSICIANS' AND NURSES' COMPLIANCE WITH TREATMENT GUIDELINES IN CANCER CARE PROGRAM

Slenker, S.E.; C.D.
Journal of Medical Education
Nov. 1985, vol. 60, p. 847-854
Treatment Guidelines

BC0130 BETTER BREAST EXAMS
Slom, C.
Reader's Digest
July 1991, vol. 139, n. n831, p. 23(1)

BC0131 BENIGN-LUMP WARNING
Squires, S.
Ladies' Home Journal
June 1992, vol. 109, n. n6, p. 50(1)
Hyperplasia

BC0132 SYNCHRONY OF MALIGNANT LYMPHOMA AND BREAST CANCER
Stierer, M. ; R.
The Journal of the American Medical Association
June 6, 1990, vol. 263, n. n21, p. 2922(2)
Malignant Lymphoma

BC0133 SCREENING MAMMOGRAPHY: BREAST CANCER DIAGNOSIS IN ASYMPTOMATIC WOMEN
Svane, G.
1993
Mammography

BC0134 PATHOLOGIC CORRELATION IN MAMMOGRAPHICALLY DIRECTED BREAST BIOPSIES
Symonds, D.A.
The Journal of the American Medical Association
Feb. 19, 1992, vol. 267, n. n7, p. 927(1)
Biopsies

BC0135 BREAST CANCER RISK AND PARTICIPATION IN MAMMOGRAPHIC SCREENING
Taplin, S.; C.
American Journal of Public Health
Nov. 1989, vol. 79, p. 1494-1498
Mammography

BC0136 WOMEN BEWARE OF BREAST CANCER
Tevis, C.
Successful Farming
Oct. 1989, vol. 87, n. n11, p. 72(1)

BC0137 BREAST CANCER TRIALS: A PATIENT'S VIEWPOINT
Thronton, H.M.
The Lancet
Jan. 4, 1992, vol. 339, n. n8784, p. 44(2)
Radiotherapy

BC0138 A DEBATE OVER EARLY CANCER DETECTION
Underwood, N.
Maclean's
Jan. 27, 1986, vol. 99, p. 49(1)
Malpractice
Anthony Miller

BC0139 QUANTITATIVE CYTO- AND HISTOPROGNOSIS IN BREAST CANCER
van Diest, P.J.
1992, vol. X, p. 211
Cyto- and Histoprognosis

BC0140 NEU-PROTEIN OVEREXPRESSION IN BREAST CANCER: ASSOCIATION WITH COMEDO-TYPE DUCTAL CARCINOMA IN SITU AND LIMITED PROGNOSTIC VALUE IN STAGE II BREAST CANCER

Vijver, M.J.; J.L.
The New England Journal of Medicine
Nov. 10, 1988, vol. 319, n. n19, p. 1239(7)
Diagnostic immunohistochemistry; carcinogenesis
Immunoprecipitation of Neu protein from metabolically labeled SKBR-3 cells. Neu-membrane stain vs path characteristics of pts with stagesII cancer. Actuarial curves for disease-free survival and overall survival. Neu-membrane staining vs path characteristics with ductal cancer in situ.

BC0141 SCREENING MAMMOGRAPHY

VomLehn, W.O.;
The Journal of the American Medical Association
Jan. 2, 1991, vol. 265, n. n1, p. 27(2)
Medical screening
Percentage of respondents knowledgeable about factors influencing cancer. (table)

BC0142 MY BREAST: ONE WOMAN'S CANCER STORY

Wadler, J.
New York
Apr. 13, 1992, vol. 25, n. n15, p. 36(12)
Diagnosis; Fibrocystic disease; Mastectomy

BC0143 SORTING THROUGH THE NUMBERS

Walsh, J.
Vogue
Oct. 1992, vol. 182, n. n10, p. 214(4)

BC0144 MAMMOGRAPHY: WHO NEEDS IT?

Weber, M.
Vogue
Jan. 1989, vol. 179, n. n1, p. 114(1)
Mammography

BC0145 BREAST CANCER: EARLIER DIAGNOSES AND NEW ATTITUDES

Weinhouse, B.
Ladies' Home Journal
Oct. 1987, vol. 104, p. 112(1)
Diagnosis

BC0146 MAMMOGRAM MADNESS

Weinhouse, B. and
Harper's Bazaar
Nov. 1991, vol. 124, n. n3359, p. 121(2)
Mammograms

BC0147 PET SCAN SPOTS BREAST-CANCER RECEPTORS

Weiss, R.
Science News
Oct. 29, 1988, vol. 134, n. n18, p. 276(1)
Tomography

BC0148 MARROW CULTURE AIDS IN CANCER PREDICTION

Weiss, R.
Science News
June 2, 1990, vol. 137, n. n22, p. 341(1)
Marrow Culture Aids

BC0149 BREAST CANCER

Weiss, R.
American Health
Sept. 1992, vol. 11, n. n7, p. 49(9)
Risk factors

BC0150 CONFRONTING BREAST CANCER: NEW OPTIONS IN DETECTION AND TREATMENT

Weitzman, S.
1986, vol. XVIII, p. 264

BC0151 STAGE AT DIAGNOSIS IN BREAST CANCER: RACE AND SOCIOECONOMIC FACTORS

Wells, B.L. and
American Journal of Public Health
Oct. 1992, vol. 82, p. 1383-1385
Diagnosis; Race; Socioeconomic Factors

BC0152 THE GOOD NEWS ABOUT BREAST CANCER; CHANGE IN DIET, NEW EARLY-DETECTION TECHNIQUES, AND REGULAR SELF-EXAMINATION CAN TURN THE STATISTICS AROUND

Wenger, L.
Weight Watchers
Mar. 1986, vol. 19, p. 64(5)
Women

BC0153 AGAINST MINIMALISM IN BREAST CANCER FOLLOW-UP

Wertheimer, M.D.
The Journal of the American Medical Association
Jan. 16, 1991, vol. 265, n. n3, p. 396(2)

Although steps have been taken to improve methods of early detection and treatment of breast cancer, the disease remains the most common female cancer and a leading cause of death. Financial limits threaten to reduce the diagnostic and therapeutic gains that have been made, as funds for mammography and research become increasingly restricted. An article in the January 16, 1991 issue of The Journal of the American Medical Association maintains the position that follow-up of patients with Stage I or II breast cancer is expensive and unlikely to lead to improved survival. Several points made in this article are questionable. In contrast with the recommendations in this report, surveillance should be maintained for its potential to improve survival and the quality of life of patients. Patients' psychological adjustment to their disease can be monitored at follow-up, as well as their overall health and the possible development of additional primary tumors. Survival advantages have been shown when asymptomatic breast cancer recurrences have been detected, and although 60 percent of metastases (spread to other organs) are discovered by patients, the rest are detected at follow-up examination. Early treatment of very small metastases is more effective than treatment of larger tumors, and usually employs approaches that are less damaging to other organ systems. Follow-up appointments with the cancer physician play an important role in the patient's life; such appointments are rarely missed. Another argument expressed in the report that cannot be supported is how money saved on follow-up might be spent (on more mammographic screening). The US health care system does not rationally set priorities or shift resources: money saved is not money more wisely spent. Better post treatment tests are needed, but cancer patients deserve and should receive intensive physician attention. (Consumer Summary produced by Reliance Medical Information. Inc.)

BC0154 PROGRESS AGAINST BREAST CANCER
Willis, J.
FDA Consumer
May 1986, vol. 20, p. 6(6)
Mastectomy
Types of mammography. Mean exposure in roentgens. Breast self-examination.

BC0155 NEW BREAST TESTS
Winter, R.
Harper's Bazaar
Apr. 1985, p. 44(2)
Monoclonal antibodies--usage; estrogen

BC0156 WHY WOMEN SHUN BREAST X-RAY EXAMS
Wood, J.
Modern Maturity
June-July 1987, vol. 30, p. 85(1)
Mammography

BC0157 BETTER TREATMENT FOR BREAST CANCER
Young, S.
Glamour
Aug. 1992, vol. 90, n. n8, p. 35(1)

BC0158 BETTER BREAST TEST
Zonis, N.
Ladies' Home Journal
Mar. 1992, vol. 109, n. n3, p. 54(1)

BC0159 ORAL CONTRACEPTIVES: NO LINK TO BREAST CANCER
USA Today
Oct. 1985, vol. 114, p. 8(1)
Oral Contraceptives

BC0160 GOOD NEWS ABOUT CANCER AND THE PILL
Newsweek
Aug. 25, 1986, vol. 108, p. 55(1)
Oral contraceptives

BC0161 PREVENTING RECURRENCE OF BREAST CANCER
USA Today
Feb. 1987, vol. 115, p. 7(1)
Tamoxifen; antineoplastic agents

BC0162 DRINKING AND BREAST CANCER
Newsweek
May 18, 1987, vol. 109, p. 73(1)
Alcohol
Doses may hurt.

BC0163 THE FUZZY LINK WITH CANCER
Economist
May 23, 1987, vol. 303, p. 92(1)

BC0164 FEMALE TROUBLE
Scientific American
July 1987, vol. 257, p. 24(2)
Women

BC0165 ALCOHOL AND BREAST CANCER
The Harvard Medical School Health Letter
July 1987, vol. 12, p. 1(2)
Cocarcinogens

BC0166 HOW STRONG IS THE ALCOHOL-BREAST CANCER LINK?
Glamour
Oct. 1987, vol. 85, p. 86(2)
Alcohol

BC0167 CANCER
USA Today
Feb. 1988, vol. 116, n. n2513, p. 5(1)

BC0168 BREASTS: IMPLANT RISK?
Vogue
Apr. 1988, vol. 178, n. n4, p. 382(1)
American Society of Plastic and Reconstructive Surgeons

BC0169 PROLACTIN A CANCER RISK?
Science News
July 9,1988, vol. 134, n. n2, p. 52(9)
Carcinogens

BC0170 ALCOHOL AND BREAST CANCER
Prevention
Nov. 1988, vol. 40, n. n11, p. 11(2)
Alcohol

BC0171 SILICONE GEL BREAST IMPLANTS: DO THEY CAUSE CANCER? WE BELIEVE NOT
Mayo Clinic Health Letter
Jan. 1989, vol. 7, n. n1, p. 8(1)
Mammaplasty

BC0172 ALCOHOL CONSUMPTION AND BREAST CANCER IN THE EPIDEMIOLOGICAL FOLLOW-UP STUDY OF THE FIRST NATIONAL HEALTH AND NUTRITION EXAMINATION SURVEY
The New England Journal of Medicine
May 7, 1987, vol. 316, p. 1169-1173
Alcohol

BC0173 BREAST CANCER
American Journal of Epidemiology
June 1990, vol. 131, p. 961-986
Medical screening

BC0174 BREAST CANCER BEFORE AGE 45 AND ORAL CONTRACEPTIVE USE: NEW FINDINGS
American Journal of Epidemiology
Feb. 1989, vol. 129, p. 269-280
Oral Contraceptives

BC0175 BREAST CANCER IN MEN: RISK FACTORS WITH HORMONAL IMPLICATIONS
American Journal of Epidemiology
Apr. 1992, vol. 135, p. 734-748
Hormonal Factors

BC0176 BREAST CANCER IN RELATION TO EARLY USE OF ORAL CONTRACEPTIVES: NO EVIDENCE OF A LATENT EFFECT
Journal of the American Medical Association
Mar. 25, 1988, vol. 259, p. 1828-1833
Risk assessment

BC0177 CIGARETTE SMOKING AND BREAST CANCER
American Journal of Epidemiology
Apr. 1986, vol. 123, p. 614-622
Smoking

BC0178 CIGARETTE SMOKING AND BREAST CANCER: CASE-CONTROL STUDIES OF PREVALENT AND INCIDENT CANCER IN THE CANADIAN NATIONAL BREAST SCREENING STUDY
Journal of Epidemiology
Aug. 1989, vol. 130, p. 213-220
Smoking

BC0179 DIFFERENCES BETWEEN BLACK AND WHITE WOMEN WITH BREAST CANCER IN TIME FROM SYMPTOM RECOGNITION TO MEDICAL CONSULTATION
Journal of the National Cancer Institute
June 17, 1992, vol. 84, p. 938-950
Black Women

BC0180 ESTROGEN REPLACEMENT AND BREAST CANCER
American Journal of Epidemiology
Dec. 15, 1991, vol. 134, p. 1375-1401
Estrogen

BC0181 A META-ANALYSIS OF THE EFFECT OF ESTROGEN REPLACEMENT THERAPY ON THE RISK OF BREAST CANCER
Journal of the American Medical Association
Apr. 17, 1991: 1985-1990, vol. 265,
Menopause; hormones

BC0182 ORAL CONTRACEPTIVE USE AND BREAST CANCER IN YOUNG WOMEN: A JOINT NATIONAL CASE-CONTROL STUDY IN SWEDEN AND NORWAY
Lancet
Sept. 20, 1986, no. 8508, p. 650-654
Women; Oral contraceptives; Sweden

BC0183 ORAL-CONTRACEPTIVE USE AND THE RISK OF BREAST CANCER: THE CANCER AND STEROID HORMONE STUDY OF THE CENTERS FOR DISEASE CONTROL AND THE NATIONAL INSTITUTE OF CHILD HEALTH AND HUMAN DEVELOPMENT
The New England Journal of Medicine
Aug. 14, 1986, vol. 315, p. 405-411
Oral Contraceptives, Steroid Hormones

BC0184 ORAL CONTRACEPTIVES AND BREAST CANCER: A PROSPECTIVE COHORT STUDY
Journal of the American Medical Association
Jan. 3, 1986, vol. 255, p. 58-61
Oral Contraceptives,

BC0185 PATTERNS OF CARE RELATED TO AGE OF BREAST CANCER PATIENTS
Journal of the Medical Association
May 22-29, 1987, vol. 257, p. 2766-2770
Age Factors

BC0186 A PROSPECTIVE COHORT STUDY OF POSTMENOPAUSAL HORMONE USE AND RISK OF BREAST CANCER IN US WOMEN
American Journal of Epidemiology
June 1987, vol. 125, p. 939-947
Women; Hormones, Postmenopause

BC0187 PROSPECTIVE STUDY OF ESTROGEN REPLACEMENT THERAPY AND RISK OF BREAST CANCER IN POSTMENOPAUSAL WOMEN
Journal of the American Medical Association
Nov. 28, 1990, vol. 264, p. 2648-2653
Sex Hormones

BC0188 PROSPECTIVE STUDY OF RELATIVE WEIGHT, HEIGHT, AND RISK OF BREAST CANCER
Journal of the American Medical Association
Nov. 24, 1989, vol. 262, p. 2853-2858
Epidemiology

BC0189 THE RELATION BETWEEN SURVIVAL AND AGE AT DIAGNOSIS IN BREAST CANCER
The New England Journal of Medicine
Aug. 28, 1986, vol. 315, p. 559-563
Diagnosis

BC0190 RELATIVE WEIGHT AND RISK OF BREAST CANCER AMONG PREMENOPAUSAL WOMEN
American Journal of Epidemiology
Nov. 1985, vol. 122, p. 731-740
Premenopause

BC0191 THE RISK OF BREAST CANCER AFTER ESTROGEN-PROGESTIN REPLACEMENT
The New England Journal of Medicine
Aug. 3, 1989, vol. 321, p. 293-297
Menopause; hormones

BC0192 THE RISK OF BREAST CANCER IN POSTMENOPAUSAL WOMEN WHO HAVE USED ESTROGEN REPLACEMENT THERAPY
Journal of the American Medical Association
Jan. 9, 1987, vol. 257, p. 209-215
cardiovascular diseases; hormones; osteoporosis

BC0193 SOCIOECONOMIC FACTORS AND RACE IN BREAST CANCER RECURRENCE AND SURVIVAL
American Journal of Epidemiology
May 16, 1992, vol. 135, p. 609-631
Race; Socioeconomic Factors

BC0194 SYNTEX ANNUAL WOMEN'S HEALTHCARE ROUNDTABLE
Syntex Laboratories
1991, p. 253
Physical examinations; ovarian cancer; cervical cancer; gynecology; menopause

BC0195 BREAST CANCER
Washington G.A.O.
Dec. 11, 1991, p. 48

BC0196 STRESS AND BREAST CANCER
1988, vol. X, p. 219
Psychosomatic aspects

BC0197 ORAL CONTRACEPTIVES AND BREAST CANCER: THE IMPLICATIONS OF THE PRESENT FINDINGS FOR INFORMED CONSENT AND INFORMED CHOICE

1990, vol. X, p. 406
Oral contraceptives

BC0198 APPROACHES TO BREAST CANCER PREVENTION

1991, vol. X, p. 244
Prevention

BC0199 BIOCHEMISTRY OF BREAST CYST FLUID: CORRELATION WITH BREAST CANCER RISK

1990, vol. VII, p. 296
Biochemistry; Cyst Fluid

BC0200 ORAL CONTRACEPTIVES AND BREAST CANCER

Institute of Medicine

1991, vol. VIII, p. 185
Oral contraceptives

BC0201 DOES THE PILL CAUSE BREAST CANCER?

Consumer Reports

Aug. 1989, vol. 54, n. n8, p. 498(3)
Contraceptive drugs; Oral contraceptives

BC0202 ESTROGEN EFFECTS ASSESSED

Science News

Aug. 5, 1989, vol. 136, n. n6, p. 86(1)
Menopause; Osteoporosis; Hormone therapy

BC0203 ESTROGEN REPLACEMENT AND BREAST CANCER

The Harvard Medical School Health Letter

Oct. 1989, vol. 14, n. n12, p. 1(3)
Hormones

BC0204 ESTROGEN REPLACEMENT: IS THERE A LINK BETWEEN ESTROGEN REPLACEMENT THERAPY AND BREAST CANCER?

Mayo Clinic Health Letter

Nov. 1989, vol. 7, n. n11, p. 6(1)
Menopause

BC0205 LIFESAVING BREAST NEWS

Glamour

Mar. 1990, vol. 88, n. n3, p. 248(4)
Self-examination; Mammography
Average risk of developing breast cancer in a given year. (table)

BC0206 CONQUERING CANCER

Harper's Bazaar

Aug. 1990, vol. 123, n. n3344, p. 46(2)

BC0207 BREAST CANCER'S AGE LINK

In Health

Sept.-Oct. 1990, vol. 4, n. n5, p. 17(1)
Age-Related factors

BC0208 ESTROGEN REPLACEMENT THERAPY IS IT LINKED TO BREAST CANCER?

Mayo Clinic Health Letter

May 1991, vol. 9, n. n5, p. 7(1)
Estrogen Replacement Therapy

BC0209 RISKS FOR BREAST CANCER

Harvard Health Letter

May 1991, vol. 16, n. n7, p. 3(1)
Risks

BC0210 SUNLIGHT AND BREAST CANCER

Chatelaine

June 1991, vol. 64, n. n6, p. 24(1)
Vitamin D in human nutrition

BC0211 BENIGN CHANGES IN THE BREAST

Consumer Reports

June 1991, vol. 56, n. n6, p. 424(1)

BC0212 ESTROGEN REPLACEMENT THERAPY: IS IT LINKED TO BREAST CANCER?

Mayo Clinic Health Letter

May 1991, vol. 9, n. n5, p. 7(1)
Estrogen Replacement Therapy

BC0213 RISKS FOR BREAST CANCER

Harvard Health Letter

May 1991, vol. 16, n. n7, p. 3(1)
Risks

BC0214 THE ESTROGEN QUESTION: IS IT A NATURAL SUPPLEMENT OR A DANGEROUS DRUG?

Consumer Reports

Sept. 1991, vol. 56, n. n9, 587(5)
Menopause; Coronary heart disease; Osteoporosis; Uterine cancer
Comparing the risks. (graph)

BC0215 STUDY LINKS BODY SHAPE, FAMILY HISTORY OF WOMEN TO RISK OF BREAST CANCER

Jet

June 1, 1992, vol. 82, n. n6, p. 25(1)
Family History

BC0216 CANCER SCREENING INTERVENTION AMONG BLACK WOMEN IN INNER-CITY ATLANTA--DESIGN OF A STUDY

Public Health Report

July-Aug. 1992, vol. 107, p. 381-388
Atlanta; Black Women

BC0217 SYSTEMATIC TREATMENT OF EARLY BREAST CANCER BY HORMONAL, CYTOTOXIC, OR IMMUNE THERAPY: 133 RANDOMISED TRIALS INVOLVING 31,000 RECURRENCES AND 24,000 DEATHS AMONG 75,000 WOMEN

The Lancet

Jan. 4, 1992, vol. 339, n. n8784, p. 1(15)
Adjuvant treatment

Hormonal treatment of early breast cancer may reduce the rate of disease recurrence and prolong survival. Data on 133 worldwide trails of adjuvant treatment of breast cancer begun before 1985 and involving 75,000 women were reviewed. Of those women, 30,000 were participating in trials of tamoxifen, an anti-estrogen that blocks the stimulation of the tumor by estrogen. After 10 years, 58.8 percent of the women taking tamoxifen were alive compared to 52.6 percent of the control group, that is, women were not taking tamoxifen. Fifty-one percent of the women in the tamoxifen group were disease-free at 10 years compared to 44.7 percent of the control group. The data from 3,000 women enrolled in ovarian ablation trials were also reviewed. Ovarian ablation involves removing the ovaries -- which produce estrogen -- or inactivating them with radiation or drugs. In women under 50, 52.9 percent in the ovarian ablation group were alive after 15 years compared to 42.3 percent in the control group.

BC0218 RELATIVE WEIGHT, HEIGHT, AND RISK OF BREAST CANCER

Albanes, D.; C.

The Journal of the American Medical Association

June 20, 1990, vol. 263, n. n23, p. 3148(1)
Risks

Distribution of body mass index and height. (table)

BC0219 CANCER WATCH IN APRIL

Alexander, W.

Black enterprise

Apr. 1991, vol. 21, n. n9, p. 16(1)
Prostate cancer

Surviving breast and prostate cancer. (graph)

BC0220 BREAST CANCER: MOVING TOWARD PREVENTION

Allison, M.

Harvard Health Letter

Aug. 1992, vol. 17, n. n10, p. 4(3)
Tamoxifen

BC0221 AT PILL'S 30TH BIRTHDAY, BREAST CANCER QUESTION IS UNRESOLVED

Althaus, F.A. and

Family Planning Perspective

July-Aug. 1990, vol. 22, p. 173-176
Contraceptives; medical care

BC0222 RELATIVE RISK: LIVING WITH A FAMILY HISTORY OF BREAST CANCER

Baker, N.C.

1991, vol. XIV, p. 236
Hereditary Risks

BC0223 RELATIVE RISK: HOW FAMILIES FACE UP TO BREAST CANCER

Baker, N.C.

Good Housekeeping

Apr. 1991, vol. 212, n. n4, p. 96(4)
Risk

BC0224 POSTMENOPAUSAL ESTROGEN REPLACEMENT AND BREAST CANCER

Barrett-Connor,
The New England Journal of Medicine
Aug. 3, 1989, vol. 321, n. n5, p. 319(2)
Hormone therapy; Uterine Cancer; Osteoporosis
The analysis of women who had been taking estrogen for many years yielded an important finding: estradiol, the most commonly prescribed noncontraceptive form of estrogen, carried nearly double the risk of breast cancer. Evidence that estrogen increases the risk of breast cancer has been difficult to obtain. The most provocative find of the study is the fourfold increase in the risk of breast cancer in women after more than four years of use of estrogen and a progestin. The addition of a progestin to estrogen is widely recommended for long-term use on the grounds that this combination is necessary to prevent endometrial hyperplasia and uterine cancer. A possibly increased risk of breast cancer in women receiving postmenopausal hormone replacement must be considered in the risk-benefit equation of such treatment.

BC0225 RISK OF BREAST CANCER AFTER ESTROGEN AND ESTROGEN-PROGESTIN REPLACEMENT

Bergkvist, L.;
The New England Journal of Medicine
Aug. 3, 1989, vol. 321, n. n5, p. 293(5)
Hormone therapy
The risk of breast cancer after non-contraceptive treatment with estrogen was examined. There is convincing evidence that hormones produced in the body are involved in the development of breast cancer. The aim of the study was to analyze the risk of breast cancer after treatment with estrogens and combinations of estrogen and progestin in a large population-based cohort. The researchers noted a ten percent increase in the relative risk of breast cancer in women for whom estrogens were prescribed for symptoms of menopause. The risk increased with increasing duration of treatment. The type of estrogen used and the presence of progestin affected the risk of breast cancer. The addition of progestin offered no protection against the development of breast cancer, which raised the important concern about the long-term treatment with a combination of estrogens and progestins that has been proposed for widespread use as prophylaxis against osteoporosis in menopausal women. Observed and expected breast cancer, duration of estrogen treatment. (table) Relative risk of breast cancer, different treatment regimens. (table) Observed and expected breast cancer, duration and type of estrogen treatment. (table)

BC0226 BREAST AUGMENTATION: A RISK FACTOR FOR BREAST CANCER?

Berkel, H.; D.C.
The New England Journal of Medicine
June 18, 1992, vol. 326, n. n25, p. 1649(5)
Silicones in medicine; Breast implants
Silicon breast implants may not increase a woman's risk of developing breast cancer. Concern has arisen that women who have silicon or polyurethane breast implants may have a higher risk of developing breast cancer than other women. A comparison of 11,676 women who received silicone breast implants to 13,557 women who were diagnosed with breast cancer found that 41 women developed breast cancer after undergoing breast augmentation surgery, which was almost half the expected number. Eighty-six percent of the women in the implant group were under 40-years-old, but 91.6 percent of those in the breast cancer group were over 40-years-old at the time of diagnosis. Women who received breast implants were followed for an average of 10.2 years, and the average length of time between breast augmentation surgery and diagnosis with breast cancer was 7.5 years.

BC0227 BREAST CANCER: THE ALCOHOL LINK

Blooston, G.
Saavy
Aug. 1988, vol. 9, n. n8, p. 14(1)
Alcohol

BC0228 CAN SEX HANGUPS CAUSE BREAST CANCER?

Boyd, P.
Harper's Bazaar
Apr. 1985, p. 44(2)
Sex (psychology); Personality
Relative risks of breast cancer

BC0229 ESTROGEN REPLACEMENT THERAPY AND RISK OF BREAST CANCER

Bush, T.L.; K.
The Journal of the American Medical Association
Sept. 11, 1991, vol. 266, n. n10, p. 1357(2)
Estrogen Repalcement Therapy

BC0230 RU 486 TAKES ON BREAST CANCER; TESTS UNDER WAY IN U.S. AND FRANCE

Carpi, J.
American Health
Oct. 1990, vol. 9, n. n8, p. 10(1)
RU 486; France

BC0231 AN OUNCE OF PREVENTION

Chisholm, P.
Maclean's
Mar. 30, 1992, vol. 105, n. n13, p. 42(2)
Tamoxifen; Low-fat diet

BC0232 A SCARE FOR PILL USERS: IS THERE A CANCER LINK?

Cowley, G.
Newsweek
Jan. 16, 1989, vol. 113, n. n3, p. 62(1)
Oral contraceptives; drugs

BC0233 CAN SUNSHINE SAVE YOUR LIFE?
Cowley, G.
Newsweek
Dec. 30, 1991, vol. 118, n. n27, p. 56(1)
Vitamin D; Solar radiation

BC0234 IN PURSUIT OF A TERRIBLE KILLER: BETTER TREATMENTS, BUT PREVENTION IS STILL A DREAM
Cowley, G.; M.
Newsweek
Dec. 10, 1990, vol. 116, n. n24, p. 66(3)
Tumors; Mastectomy; Drug therapy; Chemotherapy; Bone marrow
Breast cancer: incidence vs. mortality. (graph) TRAM flap procedure. (chart)

BC0235 PILL CLEARED OF BREAST CANCER ROLE
Davis, L.
Science News
Aug. 16, 1986, vol. 130, p. 100(2)
Carcinogens; Women

BC0236 THE IMPLANT PANIC
Davis, L.
Vogue
May 1992, vol. 182, n. n5, p. 166(3)
Silicones in surgery

BC0237 CHOLESTEROL-CANCER CLUES
Decker, C.
Science News
Mar. 31, 1990, vol. 137, n. n13, p. 198(1)
High density lipoproteins

BC0238 ESTROGEN REPLACEMENT THERAPY AND RISK OF BREAST CANCER
Dupont, W.D.;
The Journal of the American Medical Association
Apr. 10, 1991, vol. 265, n. n14, p. 1824(2)
Hormone therapy

BC0239 IF IT RUNS IN YOUR FAMILY: BREAST CANCER: REDUCING YOUR RISK
Eades, M.D.
1991, vol. XIV, p. 177
Hereditary Risks

BC0240 THE PILL AND BREAST CANCER
Edwards, D.D.
Science News
Nov. 9, 1985, vol. 128, p. 293(1)
Oral contraceptives

BC0241 ALCOHOL-BREAST CANCER LINK
Edwards, D.D.
Science News
May 9, 1987, vol. 131, p. 292(1)
Alcohol

BC0242 BREAST CANCER'S LINK TO ALCOHOL ASSAILED
Edwards, D.D.
Science News
May 28, 1988, vol .133, n. n22, p. 343(1)
Alcohol

BC0243 THE DISEASE WOMEN FEAR MOST
Englebardt, S.L.
Reader's Digest
Jan. 1989, vol. 134, n. n801, p. 61(3)

BC0244 BLOCKING BREAST CANCER: DO FAULTY ESTROGEN RECEPTORS MAKE A MEANER, TOUGHER TUMOR?
Fackelmann, K.A.
Science News
May 12, 1990, vol. 137, n. n19, p. 296(2)
Tamoxifen; Chemotherapy

BC0245 CABBAGE CHEMICAL MAY BAR BREAST CANCER
Fackelmann, K.A.
Science News
June 16, 1990, vol. 137, n. n24, p. 375(1)
Brassica; Indole

BC0246 PREVENTIVE TAMOXIFEN: SAFE SO FAR
Fackelmann, K.A.
Science News
Apr. 6, 1991, vol. 139, n. n14, p. 222(1)
Antineoplastic agents

BC0247 MALE CANCERS RAISE WOMEN'S BREAST RISKS
Fackelmann, K.A.
Science News
Aug. 8, 1992, vol. 142, n. n6, p. 85(1)
Male Cancers

BC0248 LATE-STAGE DIAGNOSIS OF BREAST CANCER IN WOMEN OF LOWER SOCIOECONOMIC STATUS: PUBLIC HEALTH IMPLICATIONS
Farley, T.A. and
American Journal of Public Health
Nov. 1989, vol. 79, p. 1508-1512
Women

BC0249 BEATING BREAST CANCER
Gorman, C.
Time
Jan. 13, 1992, vol. 139, n. n2, p. 50(1)

BC0250 ALCOHOL AND BREAST CANCER
Graham, S.
The New England Journal of Medicine
May 7, 1987, vol. 316, p. 1211(3)
Alcohol

BC0251 HETEROGENEITY OF BREAST CANCER RISK IN FAMILIES OF YOUNG BREAST CANCER PATIENTS AND CONTROLS
Grossbart-Schwar
American Journal of Epidemiology
Dec. 1, 1991, vol. 134, p. 1325-1334

BC0252 WHERE'S YOUR FAT?
Gutfield, G.; M.
Prevention
Mar. 1991, vol. 43, n. n3, p. 15(2)
Adipose tissues

BC0253 RU 486: MORE THAN AN ABORTION PILL

Hamilton, D.P.
Technology Review
May-June 1990, vol. 93, n. n4, p. 18(2)
Pro-life movement; Mifepristone
Etienne-Emile Baulieu. (portrait)

BC0254 BREAST CANCER AND ALCOHOL CONSUMPTION; A STUDY IN WEAK ASSOCIATIONS

Harris, R.E. and
JAMA: The Journal of the American Medical Association
May, 20, 1988, vol. 259, n. n19, p. 2867(5)
Alcohol
Drinking and smoking by age and other features of breast cancer patients. Characteristics of the lean subgroup of breast cancer cases. Odds ratios of breast cancer for diff. levels of alcohol consumption. Frequency distribution for nulliparity and age at 1st pregnancy. Recent published studies of alcohol and breast cancer.

BC0255 CANCER: BEATING THE ODDS

Heller, L.J.
Chatelaine
May 1990, vol. 63, n. n5, p. 113(7)
Colorectal cancer; Uterine cancer; Lymphomas
5 common cancers among women. (table)

BC0256 WHAT'S BEST FOR BREASTS?

Henig, R.M.
American Health
Apr. 1988, vol. 7, n. n3, p. 50(8)

BC0257 THE POSTMENOPAUSAL ESTROGEN/ BREAST CANCER CONTROVERSY

Henrich, J.B.
Journal of the American Medical Association
Oct. 14, 1992, vol. 268, p. 1900-1902
Cancer research; Sex hormones

BC0258 BREAST CANCER; RISK FACTORS AND GUIDE FOR WOMEN

Holleb, A.I.
Newsweek
May 30, 1988, vol. 111, n. n22, p. s18(1)
Risk Factors

BC0259 JEAN'S WAY

Humphry, D.
1986, p. 152

BC0260 WITH SURVIVAL RATES UNCHANGING AND MORE WOMEN DIAGNOSED EVERY YEAR, BREAST CANCER PREVENTION IS THE NEXT FRONTIER

Ince, S.
Vogue
Oct. 1990, vol. 180, n. n10, p. 278(5)
Tamoxifen

BC0261 WEIGHING THE EVIDENCE ON THE PILL AND BREAST CANCER

Johnson, J.H.
Family Planning Perspectives
Mar.-Apr. 1989, vol. 21, p. 89-92
Contraceptives

BC0262 DOES ALCOHOL INCREASE RISK OF BREAST CANCER?
Kaplan, J.
Vogue
Nov. 1987, vol. 177, n. n11, p. 174(1)
Alcohol

BC0263 UNDERSTANDING BREAST CANCER RISK
Kelly, P.T.
1991, vol. IX, p. 157
Risks

BC0264 BREAST CANCER AND OVARIAN CANCER: BEATING THE ODDS
Kemeny, M.M.
1992, p. 216
Ovarian Cancer

BC0265 WHO SHOULD STOP USING THE PILL? WHAT YOU MUST KNOW NOW
Kolata, G.
Glamour
May 1989, vol. 87, n. n5, p. 250(6)
Oral contraceptives

BC0266 A PROSPECTIVE STUDY OF REPRODUCTIVE FACTORS AND BREAST CANCER
Kvale, G.; I. Heuch;
American Journal of Epidemiology
Nov. 1987, vol. 126, p. 831-850
Pregnancy

BC0267 DO YOU HAVE A HIDDEN DISEASE?
Lake, A.
Woman's Day
June 2, 1992, p. 42(3)
Heart disease; Colorectal cancer; Ovarian cancer; Diabetes; Hypertension; Osteoporosis; Melanoma

BC0268 THE BREAST CANCER EPIDEMIC
Laurence, L.
McCall's
Nov. 1991, vol. 55, n. n11, p. 12(1)
Epidemics

BC0269 BREAST CANCER
Laurence, L.
Working Woman
Sept. 1992, vol. 17, n. n9, p. 91(3)

BC0270 VANADIUM AND CANCER
Lawren, B.
Omni
Nov. 1986, vol. 9, p. 52(1)
Vanadium

BC0271 SHOULD WOMEN DRINK LESS? NEW STUDIES LINK ALCOHOL CONSUMPTION TO BREAST
Lemonick, M.D.
Time
May 18, 1987, vol. 129, p. 66(1)
Infertility

BC0272 LIGHT ON BREAST CANCER

Lerch, S.

American Health

May 1991, vol. 10, n. n4, p. 86(2)
Ultraviolet radiation; Vitamin D deficiency

BC0273 LIGHT ON BREAST CANCER

Lerch, S.

American Health

May 1991, vol. 10, n, n4, p. 86(2)
Ultraviolet radiation; Vitamin D deficiency

BC0274 PREDICTING THE RISK

Lippert, J.

Weight Watchers

Apr. 1991, vol. 24, n. n4, p. 16(2)
Risk

BC0275 WOMEN'S HEALTH UPDATE

Lippert, J.

Ladies' Home Journal

Jan. 1992, vol. 109, n. n1, p. 68(2)
Menopause; Estrogen; Osteoporosis

BC0276 A PROSPECTIVE STUDY OF BENIGN BREAST DISEASE AND THE RISK OF BREAST CANCER

London, S.J.; J.L.

The Journal of the American Medical Association

Feb. 19, 1992, vol. 267, n. n7, p. 941(4)
Risks

Women with benign breast disease may have a higher risk of developing breast cancer than women who do not. Their risk may be even higher if their breast disease consist of atypical hyperplasia and they are premenopausal. A review of breast biopsy samples from 121 women in the Nurses' Health Study who subsequently developed breast cancer showed that women who had benign breast disease without atypical hyperplasia were slightly more likely to develop breast cancer. Among women younger than 55 who had atypical hyperplasia, the risk of developing breast cancer was six times the risk in women of the same age who did not have benign breast disease. In postmenopausal women with atypical hyperplasia, the risk of developing breast cancer was twice that in women without begin breast disease.

BC0277 A META-ANALYSIS OF ALCOHOL CONSUMPTION IN RELATION TO RISK OF BREAST CANCER

Longnercker,

JAMA: The Journal of the American Medical Association

Aug. 5, 1988, vol. 260, n. n5, p. 652(5)
Alcohol

Criteria for evaluating the design and data analysis of the studies. Summary of epidemiologic studies. Pooled estimates of the effect of consuming 1 g of alcohol daily. Risk of breast cancer relative to abstainers by amt. of alcohol consumed.

BC0278 BETTER, SAFER WAYS TO PROTECT YOUR BEASTS: EARLIER-THAN-EVER DETECTION AND SOME OF THE SAME DIET AND EXERCISE CHANGES THAT PREVENT HEART DISEASE CAN HELP WARD OFF BREAST CANCER, TOO

Maleskey, G.
Prevention
May 1986, vol. 38, p. 27(6)
Exercise; Diet

BC0279 IMPROVING FREQUENCY AND PROFICIENCY OF BREAST SELF-EXAMINATION: EFFECTIVENESS OF AN EDUCATION PROGRAM

Mamon, J.A. and
American Journal of Public Health
June 1985, vol. 75, p. 618-624
Self Exmination; Education

BC0280 ESTROGEN USE LINKED TO BREAST CANCER

Marx, J.L.
Science
Aug. 11, 1989, vol. 245, n. n4918, p. 593(1)
Progestation hormones

The use of long-term estrogen replacement therapy for treatment symptoms of menopause may lead to increased risk of breast cancer, according to a new study from Sweden. Estrogen therapy has been increasingly used in the U. S. to protect against the loss of minerals in the bones (osteoporosis) and cardiovascular problems that occur following the onset of menopause. The new study links risk of breast cancer from estrogen to the length of usage. After nine years of treatment, the risk becomes statistically significant, at which point the relative risk of breast cancer is nearly doubled. This study also examines the risks of breast cancer when the regimen of estrogen replacement therapy includes the combination of progestin (progesterone) with estrogen. Physicians have suspected that this combination could be more natural, and because therapy with estrogen alone has been linked to uterine cancer, this treatment might reduce the risks. However, the findings for combined treatment suggest that it may actually increase the risk of breast cancer over the risk of treatment by estrogen alone. Many in the scientific community are not surprised by this finding because estrogen has a general growth of epithelial cells such as those found in the gland and ducts of the breast. Despite this study, opinion on estrogen use for symptoms of menopause is divided. In the absence of a definitive statement, a woman's decision regarding replacement therapy is increasingly more difficult.

BC0281 BREAST CANCER

Mason-Woods, P.
Essence
Oct. 1991, vol. 22, n. n6, p. 24(2)
Mammography; Fibrocystic disease

BC0282 UPDATE ON THE PILL

McCoy, K.
Seventeen
Oct. 1989, vol. 48, n. n10, p. 52(3)
Oral contraceptives; Contraceptive drugs

BC0283 WOMEN'S CANCERS: HOW TO PREVENT THEM, HOW TO TREAT THEM, HOW TO BEAT THEM

McGinn, K.A.

1993

BC0284 PREVENTING BREAST CANCER: WHAT'S A GIRL TO DO?

Menagh, M.

Mademoiselle

Oct. 1992, vol. 98, n. n10, p. 110(2)
Prevention

BC0285 A META-ANALYSIS OF ESTROGEN REPLACEMENT AND BREAST CANCER

Mendlovic, D.; M.

The Journal of the American Medical Association

Sept. 11, 1991, vol. 266, n. n10, p. 1358(3)
Estrogen Repalcement Therapy
Risk of breast cancer. (table)

BC0286 UPLIFTING EXPERIENCES

Miller-Kase, L.

Harper's Bazaar

May 1991, vol. 124, n. n3353, p. 161(3)
Mammaplasty; Implants, Artificial

BC0287 WOMEN'S DISEASES THAT UNNERVE MEN

Moffat, O.

Chatelaine

Oct. 1991, vol. 64, n. n10, p. 39(4)
Endometriosis

BC0288 MAN TO MAN: WHEN THE WOMEN YOU LOVE HAS BREAST CANCER

Murcia, A.

1990

BC0289 BREAST-CANCER ANSWERS: A NO-PANIC REPORT ON A VERY SCARY DISEASE

Nash, J.

Mademoiselle

May 1991, vol. 97, n. n5, p. 152(1)

BC0290 BULLETIN FROM THE BREAST-CANCER FRONT

Nash, J.

Mademoiselle

Aug. 1991, vol. 97, n. n8, p. 112(1)
Fiber in human nutrition; Melatonin; Tamoxifen; Oral contraceptives

BC0291 HOW TO STOP RUNNING SCARED FROM BREAST CANCER

Neimark, J.

Mademoiselle

Feb. 1992, vol. 98, n. n2, p. 108(4)

BC0292 WOMEN WITH DISABILITIES IN THE WORK FORCE: OUTLOOK FOR THE 1990'S

OuYang, E.R.

Harvard Women's Law Journal

Spring 1990, vol. 13, p. 13-33
Maternity leave; legal cases; sex discrimination against women; sex discrimination in employment

BC0293 CANCER RATES AND RISKS
Page, H.S. and
National Institutes of Health
1985, p. 136
Carcinogens

BC0294 YOUR BEST BREAST PROTECTION
Perlmutter, C. and
Prevention
May 1992, vol. 44, n. n5, p. 36(10)
Obesity; Estrogen; Fiber in human nutrition

BC0295 REDUCING THE RISK OF BREAST CANCER
Peterson, N.
McCalls
Sep. 1989, vol. 116, n. n12, p. 101(4)
Risks
Early detection saves lives! (graph)

BC0296 THE PILL AND BREAST CANCER: NO SIGNIFICANT RISK
Port, O.
Business Week
Aug. 25, 1986, p. 94(1)
Oral contraceptives

BC0297 TIME BOMBS IN THE BREASTS? REPORTS LINKING SOME TYPES OF SILICON IMPLANTS TO CANCER STIR UP FEARS-BUT THEY MAY TURN OUT TO BE EXAGGERATED
Purvis, A.
Time
Apr. 29, 1991, vol. 137, n. n17, p. 70(1)
Silicon Implants
Diagram of a breast with silicon implant. (chart)

BC0298 PIKE'S PILL
Radetsky, P.
Discover
May 1990, vol. 11, n. n5, p. 24(2)
Oral contraceptives; Endometrial cancer; Ovarian cancer

BC0299 BLACK-WHITE DIFFERENCES IN STAGE-SPECIFIC CANCER SURVIVAL: ANALYSIS OF SEVEN SELECTED SITES
Ragland, K.E. ; S.
American Journal of Epidemiology
Apr. 1, 1991, vol. 133, p. 672-682
Black Women

BC0300 NIPPLE FLUID FLAGS BREAST CANCER RISK
Raloff, J.
Science News
Mar. 14, 1992, vol. 141, n. n11, p. 165(1)
Medical screening

BC0301 IMPLANTS: A CONNECTION TO CANCER?
Roan, S.
Los Angeles Times
Apr. 30, 1991, p. E1-E2
Product safety

BC0302 CIGARETTE SMOKING AND BREAST CANCER
Rohan, T.E. and
American Journal of Epidemiology
Jan. 1989, vol. 129, p. 36-42
Smoking

BC0303 BREAST CANCER BULLETIN
Rohlfing, C. and
Family Circle
Apr. 1, 1992, vol. 105, n. n5, p. 52(2)
Tamoxifen

BC0304 CHALLENGING THE BREAST CANCER LEGACY: A PROGRAM OF EMOTIONAL SUPPORT AND MEDICAL CARE FOR WOMEN AT RISK
Royak-Schaler, R.
1992, vol. XVII, p. 257
Psychological aspects

BC0305 WHAT, ME WORRY? HAZARDS ARE EVERYWHERE, BUT YOU'RE PROBABLY NERVOUS ABOUT THE WRONG ONES
Russel, C.; R.
American Health
June 1990, vol. 9, n. n5, p. 44(8)
Hazardous substances; Pesticides; Pollution; Benzene; Environmentally induced diseases
How the public and EPA rate health risks. (table)

BC0306 CHANGES IN SPANISH SURNAME CANCER RATES RELATIVE TO OTHER WHITES, DENVER AREA, 1969-71 TO 1979-81
Savitz, D.A.
American Journal of Public Health
Oct. 1986, vol. 76, p. 1210-1215
Spain

BC0307 ALCOHOL CONSUMPTION AND BREAST CANCER IN THE EPIDEMIOLOGIC FOLLOW-UP STUDY OF THE FIRST NATIONAL HEALTH AND NUTRITION EXAMINATION SURVEY
Schatzkin, A.; Y.
The New England Journal of Medicine
May 7, 1987, vol. 316 p. 1169(1173)
Alcohol
Drinking relations to other risk factors for breast cancer. Breast cancer incidence rates according to level of alcohol consumption. Estimates for breast cancer according to the level of alcohol intake.

BC0308 CIGARETTE SMOKING AND BREAST CANCER: A CASE-CONTROL STUDY OF SCREENING PROGRAM PARTICIPATION
Schechter, M.T.;
American Journal of Epidemiology
Apr. 1985, vol. 121, p. 479-487
Smoking; Screening

BC0309 BREAST CANCER IN RELATION TO EARLY USE OF ORAL CONTRACEPTIVES; NO EVIDENCE OF A LATENT EFFECT

Schlesselman,
JAMA: The Journal of the American Medical Association
Mar. 25, 1988, vol. 259, n. n12, p. 1828(6)
Oral contraceptives
Characteristics of women with breast cancer and control subjects. All women: relative risk of breast cancer by duration of OC use. Parous women: relative risk of breast cancer by duration of OC use. Nulliparous women: relative risk of breast cancer-total duration of OC use. Relative risk of breast cancer in relation to time since 1st use of OCs. Relative risk and latency of some hormone-dependent cancers.

BC0310 DRINKER'S DILEMMA; RAISING A GLASS MAY RAISE YOUR RISK OF BREAST CANCER AS WELL

Schwartz, J.
Health
Oct. 1987, vol. 19, p. 24(1)
Alcohol
Alcohol raises breast cancer risk.

BC0311 SILICONE BREAST IMPLANTS

Segal, M.
FDA Consumer
June 1992, vol. 26, p. 6-9
Cosmetics; product safety

BC0312 EFFECT OF FAMILY HISTORY, BODY-FAT DISTRIBUTION, AND REPRODUCTIVE FACTORS ON THE RISK OF POSTMENOPAUSAL BREAST CANCER

Sellers, T.A.; L.H.
The New England Journal of Medicine
May 14, 1992, vol. 326, n. n20, p. 1323(7)
Adipose tissues
The risk of breast cancer associated with higher waist-to-hip ratio, fewer live-born children or older age at first pregnancy may be higher among post-menopausal women who have a family history of breast cancer than those who do not. Of 37,105 55- to 69-year-old women, 493 were diagnosed with breast cancer over a four-year period. Eighty-three patients had a family history of breast cancer and 24 did not provide this information. Higher waist-to-hip ratio (circumference of the waist divided by circumference of the hip) was associated with a higher risk of breast cancer mainly in women with a family history. Association between fewer live-born children and older age at first pregnancy and breast cancer also occurred mainly in women with a family history of cancer. There may be two types of breast cancer: one that is inherited and another that develops spontaneously. Weight, fat distribution, body mass and breast cancer may share a related genetic component.

BC0313 MARILYN QUAYLE: FAMILY, FITNESS AND A BREAST CANCER CRUSADE

SerVaas, C.
The Saturday Evening Post
Oct. 1990, vol. 262, n. n7, p. 46(10)
Qualye,Marilyn
Marilyn Quayle. (portrait)

BC0314 YOUR BEST BREAST DEFENSE: HOW TO OUTSMART BREAST CANCER

Shell, E.R.
Mademoiselle
Apr. 1987, vol. 93, p. 246(4)
Food

BC0315 THE RISKS OF RISK STUDIES: IT IS TOO EASY TO DRAW ALARMING CONCLUSIONS FROM EPIDEMIOLOGICAL REPORTS

Shell, E.R.
The Atlantic
Nov. 1987, vol. 260, n. n5, p. 114(2)
Epidemiological Studies

BC0316 A TON OF PREVENTION

Shereff, R.
Ms.
Nov. 1989, vol. 18, n. n5, p. 22(1)
Prevention

BC0317 FROM ONLY ONE DRINK A WEEK? EVEN SMALL AMOUNTS OF ALCOHOL MAY TRIGGER BREAST CANCER

Siberner, J.
U.S. News and World Report
May 18, 1987, vol. 102, p. 64(2)
Alcohol

BC0318 BREAST ASSURED

Siegel, P.M.
Harper's Bazaar
Nov. 1991, vol. 124, n. n3359, p. 120(1)
Tamoxifen

BC0319 CAN YOU RUN AWAY FROM CANCER?

Simon, H.B.
Harvard Health Letter
Mar. 1992, vol. 17, n. n5, p. 5(3)
Exercise; Colorectal cancer; Reproductive organs

BC0320 BARRIERS TO CARE: THE CASE OF BREAST CANCER

Skura, B.
Health/PAC Bulletin
Summer 1991, vol. 21, p. 29-33

BC0321 BREAST IMPLANTS: WHAT DID THE INDUSTRY KNOW, AND WHEN?

Smart, T.
Business Week
June 10, 1991, no. 3217, p. 94-95, 98
Implants

BC0322 FBD: PRECURSOR TO CANCER?

Somer, E.
Shape
Sept. 1992, vol. 12, n. n1,p. 30(1)
DBD

About 50 percent of premenopausal women have sings of fibrocystic breast disease (FBD) and it is most commonly found in women in their 40s. There is no definite link with cancer, however certain types of FBD may indicate a greater cancer risk than others.

BC0323 BREAST CANCER: MOST COMMON, MOST CURABLE

Somers, R.
USA Today
Sept. 1989, vol. 118, n. n2532, p. 49(2)
Medicine, preventive

BC0324 ORAL CONTRACEPTIVES AND BREAST CANCER IN YOUNG WOMEN

Stadel, B.V.
Lancet
Nov. 2, 1985, no. 8462, p. 970-973
Oral Contraceptives

BC0325 BREAST CANCER: A FORMULA FOR PREVENTION

Stavish, S.
American health
May 1990, vol. 9, n. n4, p. 9(2)
Prevention
Risk factor A: menarche age. (table) Risk factor B: kids, moms and sibs. (table) Risk factor C: biopsies. (table) Breast test: the 30-year risk. (table)

BC0326 A META-ANALYSIS OF THE EFFECT OF ESTROGEN REPLACEMENT THERAPY ON THE RISK OF BREAST CANCER

Steinberg, K.K.;
The Journal of the American Medical Association
Apr. 17, 1991, vol. 265, n. n15, p. 1985(6)
Estrogen Replacement Therapy
Estrogen replacement therapy relieves menopausal symptoms, slows bone loss, and may protect against heart disease and reduce overall mortality. For these reasons, there was a 43 percent increase in prescriptions filled for estrogen in the United States between 1980 and 1986, from 14 million to 20 million prescriptions. However, the relationship between estrogen replacement therapy and breast cancer is not clear, and studies have reported conflicting results. To explore this issue, data were combined from 16 studies using meta-analysis, a statistical technique. Breast cancer risk was fount to increase significantly with duration of estrogen use, beginning after five years of use.

BC0327 EXERCISE: THE EFFECTS ON CANCER AND REPRODUCTION

Tangley, L. Miller, J.A.
Bioscience
May 1988, vol. 38, n. n5, p. 321(2)
Exercise

BC0328 BLACK WOMEN AND BREAST CANCER

Taylor, P.A.
Essence
June 1986, vol. 17, p. 64(2)
Black Women

BC0329 WINE, WOMEN...AND QUESTIONS

Thompson, T.
Redbook
June 1992, vol. 179, n. n2, p. 74(4)
Alcohol

BC0330 NEW PERILS OF THE PILL?: REPORTS OF A LINK TO BREAST CANCER STIR CONFUSION AND FEAR

Toufexis, A.
Time
Jan. 16, 1989, vol. 133, n. n3, p. 73(1)
Oral contraceptives; drugs

BC0331 OLD DISEASES, NEW WORRIES: ARE YOU AT RISK?

Wasco, J.
Woman's Day
Nov. 21, 1989, p. 18(1)
Whooping cough

BC0332 PATIENTS' VIEW ON BREAST CANCER...SAFER WAY TO PREVENT BLOOD CLOTS...NEW WARNINGS FOR SMOKERS...BETTER BIRTHCONTROL TIMING

Weber, M.
Vogue
Apr. 1985, vol. 175, p. 158(1)
Mastectomy; chemotherapy; aspirin; oral contraceptives

BC0333 BREAST CANCER

Weiss, R.
American Health
Sept. 1992, vol. 11, n. n7, p. 49(9)
Risk factors

BC0334 PROJECTED CHANGES IN BREAST CANCER INCIDENCE DUE TO THE TREND TOWARD DELAYED CHILDBEARING

White, E.
American Journal of Public Health
Apr. 1987, vol. 77, p. 495-497
Childbearing

BC0335 MODERATE ALCOHOL CONSUMPTION AND THE RISK OF BREAST CANCER

Willett, WC..; M.J.
The New England Journal of Medicine
May 7, 1987, vol. 316, p. 1174(7)
Alcohol

Spearman correlation coefficients. Relation of alcohol consumption to potential risk factors for breast cancer. Relative risk of breast cancer according to level of daily alcohol intake. Age-adjusted relative risk of breast cancer to level of alcohol intake.

BC0336 THE RISK OF BREAST CANCER IN POSTMENOPAUSAL WOMEN WHO HAVE USED ESTROGEN REPLACEMENT THERAPY

Wingo, P.A.; P. M.
JAMA: The Journal of the American Medical Association
Jan. 9, 1987, vol. 257, p. 209(7)
Menopause

Characteristics of postmenopausal breast cancer cases and controls. Relative risk of breast cancer by duration of estrogen replacement therapy. Relative risk of breast cancer by latency of estrogen replacement therapy. Relative risk of breast cancer of milligram-months of oral estrogen use. Relative risk of breast cancer among women with no ovaries. Relative risk of breast cancer by duration of ERT. Relative risk of breast cancer, acc. to dosage measurements of ERT.

BC0337 HEALTH AND FITNESS '87
Winter, R.E.; R.
Newsweek
June 22, 1987, vol. 109, p. S1(32)
Food; Low-cholesterol diet
Fads and facts-nutritional quiz. Dietary fiber types and sources. Cholesterol level. Cardiac risk factor questionnaire. How to examine your breasts.

BC0338 WHAT YOUNG WOMEN WANT TO KNOW ABOUT BREAST CANCER
Woodman, S.
Glamour
Oct. 1992, vol. 90, n. n10, p. 252(7)
Tamoxifen

BC0339 MODERATE ALCOHOL CONSUMPTION AND THE RISK OF BREAST CANCER
The New England Journal of Medicine
May 7, 1987, vol. 316, p. 1174-1180
Alcohol

BC0340 BUTTER- AN ANTI-TUMOR AGENT?
Science News
May 21, 1988, vol. 133, n. n21, p. 332(1)
Butter

BC0341 BREAST CANCER: LOW-FAT FINDING
Science News
Nov. 5, 1988, vol. 134, n. n19, p. 302(1)
Nutritional aspects

BC0342 DIETARY FAT AND FIBER IN RELATION TO RISK OF BREAST CANCER: AN 8-YEAR FOLLOW-UP
Journal of the American Medical Association
Oct. 21, 1992, vol. 268, p. 2037-2044
Diet

BC0343 ANIMAL PROTEIN AND BREAST CANCER: NEW ASSOCIATION REPORTED
Prevention
Aug. 1989, vol. 41, n. n8, p. 9(2)
Nutritionally induced diseases; Low-fat diet

BC0344 SMOKING, BREAST CANCER: JURY STILL OUT
Science News
Feb. 10, 1990, vol. 137, n. n6, p. 92(1)
Estrogen

BC0345 EVEN LOW-FAT DIETS POSE FAT-LINKED RISK
Science News
Aug. 25, 1990, vol. 138, n. n8, p. 126(1)

Diet

BC0346 DIET, ALCOHOL CONSUMPTION AND REPRODUCTIVE FACTORS IN A CASE-CONTROL STUDY OF BREAST CANCER IN MOSCOW
The Journal of the American Medical Association
Oct. 16, 1991, vol. 266, n. n15, p. 2072(1)
Diet, Alcohol

BC0347 MODERATE ALCOHOL CONSUMPTION AND THE RISK OF BREAST CANCER
The New England Journal of Medicine
May 7, 1987, vol. 316, p. 1174-1180
Alcohol

BC0348 AN OUNCE OF PREVENTION
Chisholm, P.
Maclean's
Mar. 30, 1992, vol. 105, n. n13, p. 42(2)
Tamoxifen; Low-fat diet

BC0349 FAT CHANCE: PREDICTING BREAST CANCER'S COURSE
Eron, C.
Science News
Aug. 13, 1988, vol. 134, n. n7, p. 100(1)
Fat

BC0350 THE DIETARY FAT-BREAST CANCER HYPOTHESIS: IT IS REALLY ALIVE?
Evans, D.A.; D.M.
The Journal of the American Medical Association
Jan. 12, 1990, vol. 263, n. n2, p. 237(2)
Diet

BC0351 A LITTLE LESS FAT WON'T CUT CANCER RISK
Ezzell, C.
Science News
Apr. 27, 1991, vol. 139, n. n17, p. 260(1)
Colorectal cancer; Prostate cancer

BC0352 TURN APPLES INTO PEARS
Gutfield, G.
Prevention
Dec, 1991, vol. 43, n. n12, p. 9(2)
Reducing diets

BC0353 FIBER FIX: BRAN MAY CUT RISK FOR BREAST CANCER
Gutfield, G.; L.
Prevention
Mar. 1992, vol. 44, n. n3, p. 9(2)
Fiber, Diet

BC0354 CUT YOUR BREAST-CANCER RISK BY 50%: WHAT TO EAT-AND NOT TO EAT- TO STAY HEALTHY
Hermann, M.G.
Redbook
June 1991, vol. 177, n. n2, p. 121(4)
Top 20 fiber bets. (table) Low-fat dairy picks. (table) Leanest meats and more. (table) Sweet treats - nice and light. (table)

BC0355 BREAST CANCER THERAPIES WEIGHED
Holden, C.
Science News
June 29, 1990, vol. 248, n. n4963, p. 1602(1)
Therapies

BC0356 A PROSPECTIVE STUDY OF SELENIUM STATUS AND BREAST CANCER RISK

Hunter, D.J.; J.S.
The Journal of the American Medical Association
Sept. 5, 1990, vol. 264, n. n9, p. 1128(4)
Dietary Supplement

It has been claimed that low levels of selenium in the diet are associated with an increased risk of cancer, and many women take supplementary selenium in the hopes of reducing their chances of developing breast cancer. However, research reports vary in the strength of association found between selenium and cancer, and one problem in evaluating patients' levels of the element is the fact that blood concentrations vary on a short-term basis, not necessarily reflecting the person's usual selenium exposure. To learn more about this, participants (female registered nurses) in a long-term study of cancer and coronary heart disease were asked to submit a set of toenail clippings for selenium analysis in 1982. Selenium concentrations in toenails are indicative of the dietary intake of selenium. More than 62,000 women submitted toenail sets; of these, 434 developed breast cancer and met the criteria for future inclusion in the study (the 'cases'). Each woman diagnosed with breast cancer was matched for age with a cancer-free woman from the group that had contributed a toenail set. When cases and controls were compared few associated between selenium levels and cancer risk factors were found. In addition, the average levels of selenium were similar in cases and controls, as was the distribution of selenium levels. Finally, no correlations were found for prognostic factors and selenium levels. Thus, the results do not support a relationship between low selenium levels in the diets of adult women and breast cancer. (Consumer Summary produced by Reliance Medical Information, Inc.) Selenium levels in toenails and risk factors. (table) Selenium levels in toenails in cases and controls. (graph) Average selenium levels in cases and controls. (table) Relative risks for breast cancer during follow-up. (table)

BC0357 THE BREAST CANCER-DIET CONNECTION

Jaskiewicz, J. and
The Saturday Evening Post
Oct. 1990, vol. 262, n. n7, p. 54(3)
Diet

BC0358 DIETARY FAT-BREAST CANCER LINK QUESTIONED

Kolata, G.
Food

BC0359 PROSPECTIVE STUDY OF RELATIVE WEIGHT, HEIGHT, AND RISK OF BREAST CANCER

London, S.J.; G.A.
The Journal of the American Medical Association
Nov. 24, 1989, vol. 262, n. n20, p. 2853(6)
Risks
Diet and energy intake are known to be associated with the incidence of mammary tumors in laboratory animals. The role of energy balance and body weight, particularly obesity, in the incidence of breast tumor is not clearly known. However, different risk rates obtained from various countries, and from the incidence rate fluctuations of populations who move from one country to another, point to a causal or etiologic role of diet in the development of breast cancer. The height and relative weight of 15,534 women who were 30 to 44 years old at the onset of this long-term study were recorded. At the time of their inclusion into the study all participants were known to be free of breast cancer. Eight years later, 648 premenopausal and 420 postmenopausal women had developed breast cancer.

BC0360 FOOD FACTORS THAT STOP CANCER: BEST NEWS, BEST BETS

Maleskey, G.
Prevention
Oct. 1987, vol. 39, p. 88(7)
Vitamin therapy; colorectal cancer; lung cancer; mouth cancer; cervical cancer

BC0361 BETTER, SAFER WAYS TO PROTECT YOUR BEASTS: EARLIER-THAN-EVER DETECTION AND SOME OF THE SAME DIET AND EXERCISE CHANGES THAT PREVENT HEART DISEASE CAN HELP WARD OFF BREAST CANCER, TOO

Maleskey, G.
Prevention
May 1986, vol. 38, p. 27(6)
Exercise; Diet

BC0362 THIS POISON COULD BECOME A POTENT POTION AGAINST CANCER

Marbach, W.D.
Business Week
July 22, 1991, n. n3223, p. 65(1)
Selenium

BC0363 THIRD STRIKE FOR NCI BREAST CANCER STUDY

Marshall, E.
Science
Dec. 14, 1990, vol. 250, n. n4987, p. 1503(2)
Women's Health Trial; Clinical trials; Diet

The National Cancer Institute (NCI) has postponed the start of a major study relating diet and breast cancer, known as the "Women's Health Trail," due to technical and ethical criticism from the scientists at the NCI. The proposal of the trial has been rejected twice before. The study is designed to determine if women can reduce their risk of breast cancer by reducing the amcunt of fat they eat. Evidence that this is true stems from studies of Japanese women who have approximately two times the incidence of breast cancer after immigrating to Hawaii compared with those who live in Japan. Those who immigrate to North America have even higher incidence of breast cancer. It appears that the increased risk is either associated with increased fat or total calorie intake. The difference in the number of individuals developing breast cancer, colon cancer, and heart disease would be studied over 15 years. The trial is estimated to cost $107 million and involve 24,000 women. It was felt that more research must be conducted on the design of the clinical trial. Problems of the design of the study are as follows: it is thought that women will not stick to either a high-fat or low-fat diet over 15 years. It would be difficult for the participants to be objective when reporting their adherence to the diet; and it would be difficult to get poor people to change their eating habits. In addition, from an ethical standpoint, thousands of women would be used in the study, as untreated controls, and these women would not be given the best dietary counseling. They would get a pamphlet recommending that they cut their intake of fat to 30 percent of the total calories they eat. The women in the experimental arm of the study would be taught how to restrict their fat to 20 percent of their total calories intake. The National Institutes of Health have in the past been accused of conducting of this trail has angered members of Congress, especially those who are women. (Consumer Summary produced by Reliance Medical Information. Inc.)

BC0364 STUDY REFINES DIET'S LINK TO BREAST CANCER

Raloff, J.
Science News
Feb. 18, 1989, vol. 135, n. n7, p. 102(1)
Diet

BC0365 DIET AND CANCER

Raloff, J.
Science News
Feb. 10, 1990, vol. 137, n. n6, p. 84(1)
Vitamin A

BC0366 BREAST CANCER RISE: DUE TO DIETARY FATS

Raloff, J.
Science News
Apr. 21, 1990, vol. 137, n. n16, p. 245(1)
Estrogen

BC0367 WHERE THE FAT IS

Reese, D.
50 Plus
Sept. 1990, vol. 30, n. n9, p. 31(1)
Adipose tissues; Heart diseases

BC0368 BREAST CANCER PREVENTION: A CONTROVERSIAL NEW DIET PROGRAM

Rennie, S.
Ms.
Apr. 1987, vol. 15, p. 40(8)
Low-fat diet

BC0369 BREAST CANCER PREVENTION: A CONTROVERSIAL NEW DIET PROGRAM

Rennie, S.
Ms.
Apr. 1987, vol. 15, p. 40-42, 51, 86-89
Diet

BC0370 DIET IN THE ETIOLOGY OF BREAST CANCER

Rohan, T.E. and
Epidemiological Reviews
1987, vol. 9, p. 120-145
Diet

BC0371 EATING TO BEAT BREAST CANCER

Sangiorgio, M.; M.
Prevention
Dec. 1990, vol. 42, n. n12, p. 10(2)
Diet

BC0372 THE DIETARY FAT-BREAST CANCER HYPOTHESIS IS ALIVE

Schatzkin, A.; P.
The Journal of the American Medical Association
June 9, 1989, vol. 261, n. n22, p. 3284(4)
Oils and fats
It is expected that 143,000 women in the U.S. will be diagnosed each year with breast cancer, and nearly one third will die of the disease. One in 8 women will develop a cancer of the breast during her lifetime. An hypothesis that the risks of breast cancer can be reduced by restricting fat in the diet has support both in the experimental and epidemiological literature. There is new evidence in support of the hypothesis and the possibility that the reports which show no correlation may have suffered from errors of design.

BC0373 SELENIUM AND BREAST CANCER

Schrauzer, G.N.;
The Journal of the American Medical Association
Jan. 2, 1991, vol. 265, n. n1, p. 28(1)
Selenium

BC0374 PERILS OF FAT: CANCER ROLE ASSAYED

Silberner, J.
Science News
Apr. 6, 1985, Vol. 127, p. 213(1)
Obesity; colon; rectum

BC0375 DEBATE RAGES OVER BREAST CANCER STUDY

Sun, M.
Science
Jan. 1, 1988, vol. 239, n. n4835, p. 17(2)
National Cancer Institute

BC0376 BREAST CANCER STUDY VETOED

Sun, M.
Science
Jan. 15, 1988, vol. 239, n. n4837, p. 252(1)

BC0377 THE NEW SCIENCE OF PROTECTIVE NUTRITION

Vaughn, L.
Prevention
Oct. 1986, vol. 38, p. 33(7)
Cholesterol; colon; calcium; low-fat diet, osteoporosis

BC0378 EAT SMART

Webb, D.
Woman's Day
Jan. 7, 1992, p. 92(1)
Food habits; Low-fat diet

BC0379 DIETARY FAT AND THE RISK OF BREAST CANCER

Willett, W.C.; M.J.
The New England Journal of Medicine
Jan. 1, 1987, vol. 316, p. 22(7)
Food--nutritional aspects

Intake of total and saturated fat, linoleic acid and cholesterol, 4 weeks. Percentage of women with risk factors for breast cancer in first, third, fifth quintile. Age-adjusted relative risk of breast cancer, adjusted calorie intake. Age-adjusted relative risk of breast cancer, unadjusted calorie intake.

BC0380 HEALTH AND FITNESS '87

Winter, R.E.; R.
Newsweek
June 22, 1987, vol. 109, p. S1(32)
Food; Low-cholesterol diet

Fads and facts-nutritional quiz. Dietary fiber types and sources. Cholesterol level. Cardiac risk factor questionnaire. How to examine your breasts.

BC0381 HER SOUL BENEATH THE BONE: WOMEN'S POETRY ON BREAST CANCER

1988, vol. XXII, p. 78

BC0382 BREAST CANCER: TEMPERING THE TRAUMA

U.S. News and World Report
Apr. 10, 1989, vol. 106, n. n14, p. 17(1)

BC0383 DISEASE AND DENIAL

Vogue
Apr. 1992, vol. 182, n. n4, p. 322(1)
Self-examination, Medical

BC0384 OLIVIA NEWTON-JOHN DISCLOSES CANCER

The New York Times Magazine
July 15, 1992, vol. 141, p. B7(N0
Newton-John, Olivia

BC0385 TREATMENT OF EARLY-STAGE BREAST CANCER

The Journal of the American Medical Association

Jan. 16, 1991, vol. 265, n. n3, p. 391(5)

A report is presented by a consensus panel of investigators, methodologists, specialists, and representatives of the public concerning optimal approaches to treating breast cancer. The panel report was formulated after the Consensus Development Conference on the Treatment of Early-Stage Breast Cancer, sponsored by the National Cancer Institute and the Office of Medical Applications of Research of the National Institutes of Health. It addressed mastectomy (removal of the breast and supporting tissues) compared with approaches that conserve breast tissue (removal of the tumor only, followed by radiation therapy); techniques of breast conserve breast tissue (removal of the tumor only, followed by radiation therapy); techniques of breast conservation; the role of adjuvant therapy (chemotherapy); the importance of prognostic factors; and future research directions. Studies with long-term follow-up have shown equivalent survival for patients choosing either mastectomy or breast conservation. Thus, the choice of a treatment is made based on other considerations, such as cosmetic results, psychosocial factors, or certain aspects of the patient's disease. Specific recommendations concerning breast conservation, with examination of lymph nodes in the armpit and subsequent radiation therapy, are presented. Although most patients without lymph node involvement are cured by either mastectomy or breast conservation treatment, chemotherapy further reduces recurrence by approximately one third. Considerable research is needed in this area, and all eligible women should be asked to participate. A good prognosis is associated with smaller tumors (especially those one centimeter or less in diameter); estrogen receptor-positive tumors (slightly better than receptor-negative tumors); lower grade cancers (a measure of aggressiveness); certain histologic types; and other factors. Future research should focus on eight areas: improving methods of rating cancer severity; developing better risk factor profiles; improving systemic chemotherapy regimens; learning more concerning the safety and efficacy of tamoxifen, a chemotherapeutic agent; assessing the quality of life for patients after cancer treatment; evaluating the efficacy of irradiation given as a 'booster'; and improving radiation therapy. Other articles concerning the treatment of breast cancer appear in the January 16, 1991 issue of The Journal of the American Medical Association. (Consumer Summary produced by Reliance Medical Information. Inc.)

BC0386 BREAST CANCER: A PATIENT GUIDE

Anderson, P.J.

1992, vol. III, p. 191

BC0387 MY SISTER'S PICTURE

Arden, C.

1986, p. 239

BC0388 A HEAVY WAIT; ONE WOMAN'S IMPATIENCE WITH BEING A PATIENT

Banks, A.

Saavy

Oct. 1987, vol. 19, p. 96(1)
Women

BC0389 MIND OVER MALADY

Barinaga, M.

Reader's Digest

Aug. 1990, vol. 137, n. n820, p. 89(2)

BC0390 BREAST CANCER: THE FACTS
Baum, M.
1988, vol. IX, p. 124

BC0391 A WOMAN'S DECISION: BREAST CARE, TREATMENT, AND RECONSTRUCTION
Berger, K.J.
1988, vol. XII, p. 266

BC0392 THE RACE IS RUN ONE STEP AT A TIME: MY PERSONAL STRUGGLE-- AND EVERYWOMAN'S GUIDE--TO TAKING CHARGE OF BREAST CANCER
Brinker, N.
1991, p. 223

BC0393 MY SISTER'S LEGACY
Brinker, N.
Ladies' Home Journal
Oct. 1990, vol. 107, n. n10, p. 156(6)
Susan Komen and Nancy Brinker. (portrait)

BC0394 GENTLE GIANTS: THE POWERFUL STORY OF ONE WOMAN'S UNCONVENTIONAL STRUGGLE AGAINST BREAST CANCER
Brohn, P.
1986, p. 178

BC0395 EHEN KREBSKRANKER FRAUEN: EINE PROSPEKTIVE UNTERSUCHUNG UBER FAMILIARE AUSWIRKUNGEN EINES MAMMAKARZINOMS
Buddeberg, C.
1985, vol. XI, p. 387
Psychological aspects

BC0396 BREAST CANCER UPDATE
Bulow-Hube, S.
Ladies' Home Journal
July 1989, vol. 106, n. n7, p. 96(2)

BC0397 CANCER IN TWO VOICES
Butler, S.
1991, vol. III, p. 183

BC0398 JOURNEY TO JUSTICE: A WOMAN'S TRUE STORY OF BREAST CANCER AND MEDICAL MALPRACTICE
Chechik, D.C.
1987, vol. XV, p. 168
Medical Malpractive

BC0399 CANCER, GOD, AND I, AND A NATURAL CURE
Cler, A.E.
1987, vol. XIII, p. 200
Natural Cures

BC0400 DYING TO LIVE
Comfort, G.
1992, vol. XII, p. 131

BC0401 J'IRAI BOIRE A LA LUMIERE
Couture-Lebel, F.
1986, p. 286

BC0402 A RACE FOR LIFE
Elliot, L.
Reader's Digest
Aug. 1985, vol. 127, p. 178(24)
Marathon running
Carol Vignal

BC0403 DO NOT GO GENTLE
Elliott, L.
The Washingtonian
June 1992, vol. 27, n. n9, p. 78(8)

BC0404 THE BIG SCARE: NANCY REAGAN'S TIME COMES
Findlay, S.
U.S. News and World Report
Oct. 26, 1987, vol. 103, p. 16(1)
Reagan, Nancy
Nancy Reagan.

BC0405 HOW I FOUGHT THE NO. 1 CANCER KILLER OF BLACK WOMEN; THE MOVING STORY OF A NURSE'S BATTLE AGAINST A MALIGNANT BREAST TUMOR
Gale, A.
Ebony
June 9, 1989, vol. 261, n. n8, p. 58(4)

BC0406 YOUNG WOMEN, CRUCIAL CHOICES
Gilbert, S.
Glamour
Nov. 1989, vol. 87, n. n11, p. 242(6)

BC0407 IN SICKNESS AND IN HEALTH
Gonzales, L.
Chicago
Aug. 1992, vol. 41, n. n8, p. 62(9)
Mastectomy

BC0408 CANCER, A SECOND FLOWERING
Graf-Ruegg, M.
1989
Psychological aspects; Art therapy

BC0409 MIND/BODY MEDICINE
Graham, B.
Vogue
Sept. 1991, vol. 181, n. n9, p. 398(2)

BC0410 INVISIBLE SCARS: A GUIDE TO COPING WITH THE EMOTIONAL IMPACT OF BREAST CANCER
Greenberg, M.
1988, vol. XIX, p. 204
Psychological aspects

BC0411 GETTING BETTER
Hargrove, A.C.
1988, p. 125

BC0412 PALOMA
Heinsohn, D.L.
Ashley Books
1987
Breast-cancer; Spain

BC0413 BREAST CANCER: THE COMPLETE GUIDE
Hirshaut, Y.
1992, vol. XIV, p. 322

BC0414 NO LESS A WOMAN: TEN WOMEN SHATTER THE MYTHS ABOUT BREAST CANCER
Hobler-Kahane, D.
1990, vol. VIII, p. 279

BC0415 LIFE WISH; THE ACTRESS AND WIFE OF SUPERSTAR CHARLES BRONSON TELLS OF HER COURAGEOUS FIGHT AGAINST BREAST CANCER
Ireland, J.
Ladies' Home Journal
Jan. 1987, vol. 104, p. 53(6)
Mastectomy
Jill Ireland and Charles Bronson

BC0416 A BATTLE WITH BREAST CANCER PUTS A STAR'S LIFE INTO FOCUS
Ireland, J.
People
Mar. 16, 1987, vol. 27, p. 57(3)
Jill Ireland

BC0417 LIFE WISH
Ireland, J.
1987, vol. VIII, p. 294

BC0418 I REFUSED TO BE A VICTIM TO CANCER
Jordan, S.
50 Plus
Apr. 1989, vol. 29, n. n4, p. 16(5)

BC0419 CANCER: FACTS VS, FEELINGS; PATIENTS ARE TREATED LIKE AIRLINE LUGGAGE: CHECKED IN, WEIGH, X-RAYED, TAGGED AND IGNORED
Kaufman, M.
Newsweek
Apr. 24, 1989, vol. 113, n. n17, p. 10(1)

BC0420 SPINNING STRAW INTO GOLD: YOUR EMOTIONAL RECOVERY FROM BREAST CANCER
Kaye, R.
1991, p. 218
Emotional Recovery

BC0421 BREAST CANCER; ANGUISH, MYSTERY AND HOPE
Kolata, G.
The New York Times Magazine
Apr. 24, 1988, vol. 137, p. 42

BC0422 BREAST CARE OPTIONS: A CANCER SPECIALIST DISCUSSES BREAST CARE OPTIONS, RISK FACTORS, AND HOW TO COPE WITH BREAST CANCER
Kuehn, P.
1986, vol. X, p. 178

BC0423 BREAST CARE OPTIONS FOR THE 1990'S
Kuehn, P.
1991, vol. VIII, p. 255

BC0424 THE ART OF HEALING
Langer, C.
Ms.
Jan.-Feb. 1989, vol. 17, n. n7-8, p. 132(2)
Diseases

BC0425 FACING BREAST CANCER WITH COURAGE; AN INTERVIEW WITH JILL IRELAND
Laughridge, J.
Harper's Bazaar
Aug. 1985, p. 196(1)
Ireland, Jill
Jill Ireland

BC0426 THE BREAST CANCER EPIDEMIC
Laurence, L.
McCall's
Nov. 1991, vol. 55, n. n11, p. 12(1)
Epididemics

BC0427 TIME FLIES WHEN YOU'RE ALIVE: A LOVE STORY
Linke, P.
1993

BC0428 A BURST OF LIGHT: ESSAYS
Lorde, A.
1988, p. 134

BC0429 DR. SUSAN LOVE'S BREAST BOOK
Love, S.M.
1990, vol. XXIII, p. 455
Love, Dr. Susan

BC0430 EXPLODING INTO LIFE
Lynch, D.
1986, p. 161

BC0431 CIVILIZATION'S CANCER
Maleskey, G.
The New York Times Magazine
Nov. 20, 1988, vol. 40, n. n12, p. 16(2)

BC0432 "I FEEL VERY LUCKY!" KATE JACKSON ON HER FRIGHTENING BATTLE WITH BREAST CANCER
McElwaine, S.
Redbook
Mar. 1991, vol. 176, n. n4, p. 36(2)
Mastectomy
Kate Jackson. (portrait)

BC0433 WOMEN'S CANCERS: HOW TO PREVENT THEM, HOW TO TREAT THEM, HOW TO BEAT THEM
McGinn, K.A.
1993

BC0434 IF YOU FIND A LUMP IN YOUR BREAST
McLean, M.
1985, p. 85
Lumps

BC0435 MAN TO MAN: WHEN THE WOMEN YOU LOVE HAS BREAST CANCER
Murcia, A.
1989, vol. XII, p. 220

BC0436 HOW TO STOP RUNNING SCARED FROM BREAST CANCER
Neimark, J.
Mademoiselle
Feb. 1992, vol. 98, n. n2, p. 108(4)

BC0437 JUST IN TIME
Newman, P.
Cosmopolitan
Nov. 1988, vol. 205, n. n5, p. 260(5)

BC0438 BREAST CANCER IN THE LIFE COURSE: WOMEN'S EXPERIENCES
Oktay, J.S.
Springer Series on Social Work
1991, vol. X, p. 220

BC0439 OF TEARS AND TRIUMPHS
Photopulos, G.
1988, vol. XIV, p. 204

BC0440 MARY BETH DOLIN'S COURAGEOUS FIGHT AGAINST CANCER
Prodanou, A.
Chatelaine
Sept. 1985, vol. 58, p. 54(4)
Dolin, Mary Beth
Mary Beth Dolin

BC0441 THE C LIST
Rapoport, N.
The New York Times Magazine
Sept. 8, 1991, vol. 140, p. 22

BC0442 PSYCHOLOGICAL ASPECTS OF EARLY BREAST CANCER
Ray, C.
Springer-Verlag
1985, p. 133
Stress; Psychotherapy

BC0443 ARE WE WINNING THE WAR AGAINST CANCER?
Rock, A.; K. Casey;
Ladies' Home Journal
Sept. 1991, vol. 108, n. n9, p. 167(12)
Medical research
Betty Ford and Ann Jillian. (portrait) Marilyn Quayle. (portrait)
Incidence rates. (graph) Death rates. (graph)

BC0444 BREAST CANCER: FACING THE FEAR
Royak-Schaler, R.
Glamour
Mar. 1992, vol. 90, n. n3, p. 244(6)

BC0445 MOTHER'S BREAST
Schrieberg, D.
Mother Jones
Nov.-Dec. 1992, vol. 17, p. 33-39, 69-72

BC0446 PSYCHISCHE BEWALTIGUNGSSTRATEGIAN BEI BRUSTKREBSPATIENTINNEN
Schroder, A.
Series VI, Psychology
1985, vol. 160, p. 201
Women--Psychology

BC0447 EVERY WOMAN'S GUIDE TO BREAST CANCER: PREVENTION, TREATMENT, RECOVERY
Seltzer, V.L.
1987, vol. XIII, p. 209

BC0448 THE JOURNEY BEYOND BREAST CANCER: FROM THE PERSONAL TO THE POLITICAL: TAKING AN ACTIVE ROLE IN PREVENTION, DIAGNOSIS, AND YOUR OWN HEALING
Soffa, V.M.
1992

BC0449 MAKE SURE YOU DO NOT HAVE BREAST CANCER
Strax, P.
1991, vol. XIV, p. 236

BC0450 OVERCOMING BREAST CANCER
Subak-Sharpe,
1987, vol. X, P. 180

BC0451 LIVING WITH BREAST CANCER AND MASTECTOMY: A SELF-HELP GUIDE
Tarrier, N.
1987, p. 128
Psychological Aspects

BC0452 MY BREAST: ONE WOMAN'S CANCER STORY
Wadler, J.
1992

BC0453 MY BREAST: ONE WOMAN'S CANCER STORY
Wadler, J.
New York
Apr. 20, 1992, vol. 25, n. n16, p. 48(11)
Care and treatment; Surgery

BC0454 IN GOD'S HAND: ONE WOMAN'S EXPERIENCE WITH BREAST CANCER
Wecksler, B.L.
1989, p. 102

BC0455 REFUGE: AN UNNATURAL HISTORY OF FAMILY AND PLACE
Williams, T.T.
1991, vol. XIII, p. 304

BC0456 REFUGE: AN UNNATURAL HISTORY OF FAMILY AND PLACE
Williams, T.T.
1992, vol. XVI, p. 304

BC0457 CHEMO AND LUNCH: ONE WOMAN'S TRIUMPH OVER HEREDITARY BREAST CANCER
Winn, S.
1990, p. 112
Hereditary; Chemioterapy

BC0458 SURGERY FOR BREAST CANCER: PRESERVE AND PROTECT
The Harvard Medical School Health Letter
July 1985, vol. 10, p. 2(3)
Mastectomy

BC0459 FIVE-YEAR RESULTS OF A RANDOMIZED CLINICAL TRIAL COMPARING TOTAL MASTECTOMY AND SEGMENTAL MASTECTOMY WITH OR WITHOUT RADIATION IN THE TREATMENT OF BREAST CANCER
The New England Journal of Medicine
Mar. 14, 1985, vol 312, p. 665-673
Mastectomy

BC0460 GEOGRAPHIC VARIATION IN THE USE OF BREAST-CONSERVING TREATMENT FOR BREAST CANCER
The New England Journal of Medicine
Apr. 23, 1992, vol. 326, p. 1102-1107
Surgery

BC0461 BREAST RECONSTRUCTION: A MATTER OF CHOICE
The Institute
1990, p. 18
Breast Reconstruction

BC0462 TEN-YEAR RESULTS OF A RANDOMIZED CLINICAL TRIAL COMPARING RADICAL MASTECTOMY AND TOTAL MASTECTOMY WITH OR WITHOUT RADIATION
The New England Journal of Medicine
Mar. 14, 1985, Vol. 312, p. 674-681
Mastectomy

BC0463 TEN-TEAR RESULTS OF A RANDOMIZED CLINICAL TRIAL COMPARING RADICAL MASTECTOMY AND TOTAL MASTECTOMY WITH OR WITHOUT RADIATION
The New England Journal of Medicine
Mar. 14, 1985, vol. 312, p. 674-681
Mastectomy

BC0464 SURGERY OF THE BREAST: DIAGNOSIS AND TREATMENT OF BREAST DISEASES
1986, p. 336
Surgery

BC0465 BREAST CANCER: CONSERVATIVE AND RECONSTRUCTIVE SURGERY
Brustkrebs und Brustrekonstruktion
1989, vol. XX, p. 539

BC0466 BREAST DISEASES: BREAST-CONSERVING THERAPY, NON-EVASIVE LESIONS, MASTOPATHY
1989, vol. XVIII, p. 548
Mastopathy

BC0467 THERAPY CHOICE BENEFITS PATIENTS
USA Today
Feb. 1990, vol, 118, n. n2537, p. 3(1)

BC0468 TREATMENT OF EARLY-STAGE BREAST CANCER

The Journal of the American Medical Association

Jan. 16, 1991, vol. 265, n. n3, p. 391(5)
Early Cancer
A report is presented by a consensus panel of investigators, methodologists, specialists, and representatives of the public concerning optimal approaches to treating breast cancer. The panel report was formulated after the Consensus Development Conference on the Treatment of Early-Stage Breast Cancer, sponsored by the National Cancer Institute and the Office of Medical Applications of Research of the National Institutes of Health. It addressed mastectomy (removal of the breast and supporting tissues) compared with approaches that conserve breast tissue (removal of the tumor only, followed by radiation therapy); techniques of breast conserve breast tissue (removal of the tumor only, followed by radiation therapy); techniques of breast conservation; the role of adjuvant therapy (chemotherapy); the importance of prognostic factors; and future research directions. Studies with long-term follow-up have shown equivalent survival for patients choosing either mastectomy or breast conservation. Thus, the choice of a treatment is made based on other considerations, such as cosmetic results, psychosocial factors, or certain aspects of the patient's disease. Specific recommendations concerning breast conservation, with examination of lymph nodes in the armpit and subsequent radiation therapy, are presented. Although most patients without lymph node involvement are cured by either mastectomy or breast conservation treatment, chemotherapy further reduces recurrence by approximately one third. Considerable research is needed in this area, and all eligible women should be asked to participate. A good prognosis is associated with smaller tumors (especially those one centimeter or less in diameter); estrogen receptor-positive tumors (slightly better than receptor-negative tumors); lower grade cancers (a measure of aggressiveness); certain histologic types; and other factors. Future research should focus on eight areas: improving methods of rating cancer severity; developing better risk factor profiles; improving systemic chemotherapy regimens; learning more concerning the safety and efficacy of tamoxifen, a chemotherapeutic agent; assessing the quality of life for patients after cancer treatment; evaluating the efficacy of irradiation given as a 'booster'; and improving radiation therapy. Other articles concerning the treatment of breast cancer appear in the January 16, 1991 issue of The Journal of the American Medical Association. (Consumer Summary produced by Reliance Medical Information. Inc.)

BC0469 SAFE, BETTER BREAST SURGERY

Vogue

Feb. 1991, vol. 181, n. n2, p. 246(1)
Surgery, plastic

BC0470 BEST TIME TO BEAT BREAST CANCER?

Science News

June 8, 1991, vol. 139, n. n23, p. 365(1)

BC0471 FIGHTING CANCER: NEWS FROM THE FRONT

Vogue

Oct. 1991, vol. 181, n. n10, p. 210(1)
Menstrual cycle; Ovarian cancer

BC0472 COMBINE TREATMENTS FOR BEST RESULTS

USA Today

Oct. 1991, vol. 120, n. n2557, p. 4(1)
Mastectomy; Radiotherapy; Chemotherapy

BC0473 TIMING OF BREAST CANCER EXCISION DURING THE MENSTRUAL CYCLE INFLUENCES DURATION OF DISEASE-FREE SURVIVAL

The Journal of the American Medical Association

Dec. 18, 1991, vol. 266, n. n23, p. 3276(1)
Surgery

BC0474 TIMING CANCER SURGERY

Reader's Digest

Feb. 1992, vol. 120, n. n838, p. 24(1)
Surgery

BC0475 THE TAKE-CHARGE PATIENT

Atkins, A.

Ladies' Home Journal

Nov. 1990, vol. 107, n. n11, p. 163(6)
Menopause; Hysterectomy; Mastectomy
Hysterectomy and its possible alternatives. (table)
Hormone-replacement therapy. (table) Treating breast cancer. (table)

BC0476 A WOMAN'S DECISION: BREAST CARE, TREATMENT, AND RECONSTRUCTION

Berger, K.J.

1988, vol. XII, p. 266

BC0477 OVER-40 GOOD HEALTH AND GREAT LOOKS

Bersch, S.; R.

Harper's Bazaar

Aug. 1989, vol. 122, n. n3332, p. 132(10)

BC0478 BREAST-CANCER UPDATE

Boffey, P.M.

Reader's Digest

Aug. 1985, vol. 127, p. 18(2)
Surgery

BC0479 MASTECTOMY VS. LUMPECTOMY

Bolick, N.O.

Boston

July 1985, vol. 77, p. 134(4)
Mastectomy; Lumpectomy

BC0480 GEOGRAPHIC VARIATION IN THE USE OF BREAST-CONSERVING TREATMENT FOR BREAST CANCER

Butler-Nattinger,
The New England Journal of Medicine
Apr. 23, 1992, vol. 326, n. n17, p. 1102(6)
Mastectomy; Lumpectomy
Differences in the use of breast-conserving surgery to treat breast cancer patients in different regions of the U. S. cannot be explained by differences in hospital characteristics. Of 36,982 65- to 79-year-old female Medicare patients with breast cancer that had not spread or had spread only regionally into the lymph nodes, 12.1 percent underwent breast-conserving surgery; 87.9 percent underwent some type of total mastectomy. The percentage of women who underwent breast-conserving surgery varied from 3.5 percent in Kentucky to 21.2 percent in Massachusetts. Use of breast-conserving surgery was significantly higher in the New England and Middle Atlantic states, and significantly lower in the South Atlantic, South Central, and West North Central states. Women were more likely to undergo breast-conserving surgery in urban hospitals, in teaching hospitals, in larger hospitals and in hospitals with radiation therapy facilities, geriatric services or a cancer center. Variation in treatment of breast cancer patients in different regions remained after taking into account differences in hospital characteristics.

BC0481 VALUE OF AXILLARY DISSECTION IN ADDITION TO LUMPECTOMY AND RADIOTHERAPY IN EARLY BREAST CANCER

Cabanes, P.A.;
The Lancet
May 23, 1992, vol. 339, n. n8804, p. 1245(4)
Lymph nodes
Women with early breast cancer who have a lumpectomy may also benefit from having the lymph nodes under their arms removed, a procedure known as axillary dissection. Of 658 women with tumors less than 3 centimeters and no suspected lymph node involvement, 332 received a lumpectomy and 326 received a lumpectomy and axillary dissection. Sixty women treated with lumpectomy and axillary dissection were found to have lymph node metastases at surgery. The average follow-up for all the women was 54 months. At five years, 92.6 percent of the women who received only a lumpectomy and 96.6 percent of the women who received a lumpectomy and axillary dissection were alive. The cancer recurrence rates were similar in both groups, but cancer was less likely to recur in the lymph nodes in the women who received axillary dissection. The likelihood of preserving the breast was equally high in both groups. The women who received axillary dissection experienced no serious complications from the surgery.

BC0482 BREAST CANCER TREATMENTS

Cimons, M.; A.
50 Plus
Oct. 1990, vol. 30, n. n10, p. 44(3)
Lumpectomy; Mastectomy; Mammography

BC0483 BREAST CANCER: A KINDER CURE

Clark, M Witherspoon
Newsweek
Feb. 18, 1985, vol. 105, p. 85(1)
Mastectomy
Mastectomies: charting the change

BC0484 THE PASSION OF DOCTOR LOVE

Diamant, A.
Boston
Oct. 1988, vol. 80, n. n10, p. 162(13)
Women surgeons
Susan Love.

BC0485 DO YOU NEED THESE OPERATIONS?

Dranov, P.
Health
June 1986, vol. 18, p. 24(4)
Uterus; Tumors; Consumer protection

BC0486 BEST TIME FOR BREAST CANCER SURGERY

Fackelmann, K.A.
Science News
Apr. 11, 1992, vol. 141, n. n15, p. 239(1)
Care and treatment

BC0487 HEALING WITH LIGHT

Faivelson, S.
50 Plus
Nov. 1991, vol. 31, n. n10, p. 70(3)
Fibromas

BC0488 GEOGRAPHIC VARIATION IN THE TREATMENT OF LOCALIZED BREAST CANCER

Farrow, D.C.; W.C.
The New England Journal of Medicine
Apr. 23, 1992, vol. 326, n. n17, p. 1097(5)
Mastectomy; Lumpectomy

Use of breast-conserving surgery to treat women with breast cancer that has not spread varies among different regions of the U. S. Data from the National Cancer Institute on the types of surgery used to treat 18,399 non-Hispanic white, 324 Hispanic and 1,174 black women with breast cancer in nine different regions of the U. S. between 1983 and 1986 show variation in all age groups. The percentage of white women who had breast-conserving surgery varied from 9.2 percent in Iowa to 41.5 percent in Seattle, WA. The proportion of white women who received radiation therapy also was lowest in Iowa, and highest in Seattle, WA. The number of white women who had breast-conserving surgery and/or radiation therapy increased between 1983 and 1986, but the relative percentages of women who had these treatments in different regions remained approximately the same. Use of breast-conserving surgery to treat Hispanic and black women was approximately the same as for white women in different regions. Older women and black women in Atlanta, GA and Detroit, MI, however, were less likely than other women to receive radiation therapy after breast-conserving surgery.

BC0489 EIGHT-YEAR RESULTS OF A RANDOMIZED CLINICAL TRIAL COMPARING TOTAL MASTECTOMY AND LUMPECTOMY WITH OR WITHOUT IRRADIATION IN THE TREATMENT OF BREAST CANCER

Fisher, B.; C.
The New England Journal of Medicine
Mar. 30, 1989, vol. 320, n. n13, p. 822(7)
Radiotherapy; Lymph nodes
Lumpectomy, the surgical removal of a tumor from the breast, followed by radiation therapy, was conducted in 1,843 patients suffering from Stage I or II breast cancer. Chemotherapy was used as well in those women with cancer surrounding the nodes near the breast. Lumpectomy followed by radiation therapy resulted in a five-year survival rate of 85 percent, whereas the five-year survival rate of total mastectomy was 76 percent. At follow-up eight years after initial treatments, 90 percent of the women who underwent lumpectomy followed by irradiation were free of tumors in the same breast, while only 61 percent of patients who did not receive radiation treatment remained tumor-free. In addition, 94 percent of the patients with lymph node involvement who were treated with a combination of lumpectomy, radiation, and chemotherapy had no recurrences in the breast treated. The value of radiation therapy in reducing the recurrence of tumors following lumpectomy continues to be significant. Furthermore, the data to date continue to support breast conservation (as contrasted with total mastectomy) for patients with primary breast cancer (cancer which has not moved to other sites in the body. Distribution of patients according to treatment group. (table) Life-time table analysis: percentage who remained free of breast tumor. (graph) Disease-free survival rate and cumulative incidence of events, each group. (table) Life table analysis showing rates of disease-free survival. (graph) Comparison of 5-year life-table estimates and results. (table) Comparison of mastectomy, lumpectomy, and lumpectomy with radiation therapy. (table) Lumpectomy and lumpectomy with irradiation, according to node status. (table)

BC0490 QUALITY OF CARE

Friedell, P.E.; J.J.
The Journal of the American Medical Association
Apr. 22, 1992, vol. 267, n. n16, p. 2186(3)
Lumpectomy; Radiotherapy

BC0491 TREATMENT OPTIONS FOR BREAST CANCER-BEYOND SURVIVAL

Ganz, P.A.

The New England Journal of Medicine

Apr. 23, 1992, vol. 326, n. n17, p. 1147(3)
Mastectomy; Lumpectomy; Informed consent (Medical law)

Advances in the understanding of breast cancer have changed treatment options for women with early stage breast cancer. Many of these women can be treated with breast-conserving surgery such as a lumpectomy, quadrantectomy or partial mastectomy rather than a radical mastectomy. Two research studies found that breast-conserving surgery is used to treat woman with early-stage breast cancer most often in the Northeast U. S., least often in the Southeast U. S. and most often in the 17 states with informed consent laws. The use of breast-conserving surgery also was related to the type of hospital at which the patient was treated. These studies also found that use of breast-conserving surgery was lower in older women, and fewer older women who had breast-conserving surgery had radiation therapy. Surgeons' beliefs and practice methods, especially in providing information on treatment options, may affect the use of breast-conserving therapy. The effect of a radical mastectomy on a woman's quality of life should be weighed against the threat of cancer recurrence.

BC0492 BREAST CANCER: IMPORTANCE OF ADEQUATE SURGICAL EXCISION PRIOR TO RADIOTHERAPY IN THE LOCAL CONTROL OF BREAST CANCER IN PATIENTS TREATED CONSERVATIVELY

Ghossein, N.A.

The Journal of the American Medical Association

June 24, 1992, vol. 267, n. n26, p. 3274(1)

BC0493 IN SICKNESS AND IN HEALTH

Gonzales, L.

Chicago

Aug. 1992, vol. 41, n. n8, p. 62(9)
Mastectomy

BC0494 TREATMENT TRENDS

Gupta, E.; N.

Ladies' Home Journal

July 1989, vol. 106, n. n7, p. 98(2)
Lasers in surgery

BC0495 YOUR BREAST AND YOU: WHAT EVERY WOMAN NEEDS TO KNOW ABOUT BREAST DISEASES, BREAST CANCER, AND COSMETIC BREAST SURGERY BEFORE SHE HAS A PROBLEM

Halbert, D.S.

1985, p. 238
Gynecology

BC0496 BREAST CANCER

Hicks, N. and G.

Glamour

May 1986, vol. 84, p. 222(6)

BC0497 DIAGNOSIS: BREAST CANCER-TREATMENT: NOT NECESSARILY A MASTECTOMY

Jabs, C.

Woman's Day

Apr. 15, 1986, p. 96(2)
Mastectomy

BC0498 SPINNING STRAW INTO GOLD: YOUR EMOTIONAL RECOVERY FROM BREAST CANCER

Kaye, R.

1991, p. 218
Emotional Recovery

BC0499 "I GUESS IT'S MY TURN"; NANCY REAGAN BRAVELY ENDURES A MODIFIED RADICAL MASTECTOMY

Lamar, J.V. Jr.

Time

Oct. 26, 1987, vol. 130, p. 36(1)
Reagan, Nancy; Mastectomh
Nancy Reagan

BC0500 UNDERUTILIZATION OF BREAST-CONSERVING SURGERY AND RADIATION THERAPY AMONG WOMEN WITH STAGE I AND II BREAST CANCER

Lazovich, D.; E.

The Journal of the American Medical Association

Dec. 25, 1991, vol. 266, n. n24, p. 3433(6)
Lumpectomy

Traditionally, breast cancer was treat using the Halsted mastectomy, surgical removal of the breast, underlying chest muscles, and axillary contents. Recent research has indicated that among women with breast cancer in its early stages, conservative treatment involving only excision of the tumor and surrounding tissue followed by radiation therapy is preferable. In 1990, the National Institutes of Health (NIH) recommended conservative treatment, or breast-conserving surgery (BCS), for early-stage breast cancer. This study examined the use of BCS in women with early-stage breast cancer. Treatment data were obtained for women residing in the Seattle area who had either stage I or II breast cancer and were treated between 1983 and 1989. BCS was performed on 33.7 percent of the women. Only 25.7 percent of the women with stage II disease underwent BCS, while 42.6 percent of the women with stage I disease had BCS. BCS was most widely used in 1985, a significant difference from 1983 and 1984. Slight declines in use of BCS occurred after the peak in 1985. BCS was more likely to be used when the patients were younger, more affluent, or more educated. Between 12 and 16 percent of the patients treated with BCS were not given postoperative radiation therapy. Women not given radiation therapy tended to be older, to have stage II disease, or to live in an area without radiation therapy facilities. These results indicate that BCS (and in some cases radiation therapy) was underutilized as a treatment for early-stage breast cancer in this population. In addition, the factors associated with the use (and nonuse) of BCS do not reflect the criteria established by the National Institutes of health. (Consumer Summary produced by Reliance Medical Information. Inc.)
Characteristics of study subjects. (table) Effects of stage and time trends on use of BCS. (table) Effects of various demographic factors on use of BCS. (table) Percentages of women who underwent BCS. (graph) The risk of failure to receive radiation therapy after BCS. (table)

BC0501 CHANGING TREATMENT OF BREAST CANCER IN NEW MEXICO FROM 1969 THROUGH 1985

Mann, B.A.; J.M.
JAMA: The Journal of the American Medical Association
June 17, 1988, vol. 259, n. n23, p. 3413(5)
Surgical research

Percent of women with local-stage breast cancer. Percent of patients with local-stage breast cancer. Percent of women with regional-stage breast cancer. No, of women with local-stage breast cancer who underwent surgery.

BC0502 PROGNOSTIC FACTORS AND TREATMENT DECISIONS IN AXILLARY-NODE-NEGATIVE BREAST CANCER

McGuire, W.L.;
The New England Journal of Medicine
June 25, 1992, vol. 326, n. n26, p. 1756(6)
Tumors

Of the estimated 186,000 cases of breast cancer that will be diagnosed in 1992, two-third will be node-negative; that is, the cancer will not have spread to lymph nodes under the arm. Since 70 percent of these women can be cured without chemotherapy, this treatment should be limited to those who have a high risk of cancer recurrence. This can be determined using several prognostic factors. Several studies have shown that the smaller the tumor, the greater the long-term survival and duration of life cancer-free. Certain histologic types, such as ductal carcinoma in situ, also have a good prognosis. The presence or absence of estrogen receptors in the tumor may be useful when combined with other factors. Abnormal DNA content may or may not indicate a worse prognosis, but tumors that are actively proliferating have a worse prognosis. Excessive levels of the enzyme cathepsin D are associated with high cancer recurrence and poor survival. Once a woman's prognostic factors have been identified, treatment can be tailored accordingly.

BC0503 BREAST-CANCER TREATMENT; WHAT ARE THE PROS AND CONS OF CURRENT OPTIONS

Michaels, E.
Chatelaine
Jan. 1988, vol. 61, n. n1, p. 28(1)
Treatments

Types of mastectomy.

BC0504 THE LOWDOWN ON LUMPECTOMY: WHAT EVERY WOMAN SHOULD KNOW ABOUT THIS BREAST-SPARING CANCER TREATMENT

Michaud, E. and
Prevention
Sept. 1990, vol. 42, n. n9, p. 56(11)

BC0505 "LETS JUST HOLD HANDS"

Morganthau, T.;
Newsweek
Oct. 26, 1987, vol. 110, p. 28(2)

BC0506 AURODESK'S CEO TO TAKE MEDICAL LEAVE UNTIL MID-JULY

Morrissey, J.
PC Week
June 15, 1992, vol. 9, n. n24, 162(1)
Medical Issues

BC0507 MY LUMPECTOMY

Mosley, G.
Good Housekeeping
Apr. 1990, vol. 210, n. n4, p. 78(3)
Lumpectomy

BC0508 METASTATIC BREAST CANCER: LENGTH AND QUALITY OF LIFE

Norton, L.
The New England Journal of Medicine
Nov. 7, 1991, vol. 325, n. n19, p. 1370(2)
Metastatic Cancer

Metastatic breast cancer is incurable. When breast cancer cells have colonized other organs of the body and begun developing into secondary tumors, the only course of treatment is the palliation of symptoms. Some patients respond to hormonal treatment, and this is particularly useful since hormonal therapy does not cause many of the grave side effects of conventional chemotherapy. However, in all cases, the cancer will eventually become unresponsive, and more aggressive therapy will be needed. In the November 7, 1991 issue of The New England Journal of Medicine, researchers report that continued chemotherapeutic treatment of patients with advanced breast cancer results in a longer period of freedom from symptoms, but does not improve survival compared with interrupted treatment. In the latter case, patients are treated and observed for signs of disease progression, at which time they may receive further chemotherapy. This is important information of the practicing oncologist, who may advise women responding well to chemotherapeutic treatment that continued treatment is likely to extend period of improved quality of life. The results also indicate that women who are experiencing the more severe side effects of chemotherapy may be advised that the discontinuation of treatment will not affect their survival. The observations made in this study raise some other basic scientific questions, however. In animal studies, chemotherapeutic treatment that induces a remission almost invariably lengthens survival. The principle seems simple. If the majority of cancer cells are destroyed, the remaining few take longer to grow to extend that will kill the animal. Among human patients, however, the destruction of the majority of cancer cells often does not lengthen survival. Why this should be is not understood. One possibility is that the cancer cells remaining after chemotherapy actually grow more rapidly than they did before treatment. If this is the case, identifying the factors that alter the rates of growth of cancer cells might result in the development of improved techniques of therapy. (Consumer Summary produced by Reliance Medical Information. Inc.)

BC0509 PATHOLOGY EVALUATION OF LUMPECTOMY SPECIMEN

Oxley, D.K. and C.
The Journal of the American Medical Association
Jan. 16, 1991, vol. 265, n. n3, p. 412(1)
Lumpectomy

BC0510 STAGE I AND II BREAST CANCER: WHAT TYPE OF SURGERY

Quattlebaum, J.K.;
The Journal of the American Medical Association
Apr. 15, 1992, vol. 267, n. n15, p. 2038(2)
Surgery

BC0511 COLOR ATLAS OF MODIFIED RADICAL MASTECTOMY
Ralphs, D.
Medical Economics Books
1985, p. 64
Surgery, Radical Mastectomy

BC0512 SURGICAL PATHOLOGY OF THE BREAST
Rogers, K.
1990, p. 149
Surgical Pathology

BC0513 IT WASN'T THE END OF THE WORLD; BREAST CANCER IN THE 80'S DOESN'T HAVE TO MEAN A MASTECTOMY
Roy, A.
Working Woman
Mar. 1987, vol. 12, p. 126(5)
Mastectomy

BC0514 NONCLINICAL FACTORS ASSOCIATED WITH SURGERY RECEIVED FOR TREATMENT OF EARLY-STAGE BREAST CANCER
Satariano, E.R.;
American Journal of Public Health
Feb. 1992, vol. 82, p. 195-198
Surgery

BC0515 DR. GEORGE CRILE JR., 84, FOE OF UNNEEDED SURGERY, DIES
Saxon, W.
The New York Times
Sept. 12, 1992, vol. 141, p. 28(N) p10
Crile, Dr. George

BC0516 BREAST CANCER: WOMAN IS PARTNER IN CHOOSING TREATMENT
Segal, M.
FDA Consumer
Sept. 1991, vol. 25, n. n7, p. 18(6)
Breast implants; Mastectomy; Chemotherapy

BC0517 CANCER: A RADICAL DEPARTURE
Seligmann, J.
Newsweek
Mar. 25, 1985, vol. 105, p. 91(1)
Mastectomy
How effective is surgery that spares the breast?

BC0518 BREAST CANCER: NEW FACTS, NEW FEARS; LUMPECTOMY, THE RIGHT TO CHOOSE
Spear, R.
Ladies' Home Journal
Feb. 1988, vol. 105, n. n2, p. 71(4)
Mastectomy

BC0519 PSYCHOLOGICAL OUTCOME OF LUMPECTOMY VERSUS MASTECTOMY IN THE TREATMENT OF BREAST CANCER
Steinberg, M.D.;
American Journal of Psychiatry
Jan. 1985, vol. 142, p. 34-39
Radiotherapy; mental health
B

BC0520 CONSERVATIVE SURGERY AND RADIATION FOR INTRADUCTAL BREAST CARCINOMA
Valenti, F.D.; W.T.
The Journal of the American Medical Association
July 8, 1992, vol. 268, n. n2, p. 266(1)
Surgery, Conservative

BC0521 MY BREAST: ONE WOMAN'S CANCER STORY
Wadler, J.
New York
Apr. 13, 1992, vol. 25, n. n15, p. 36(12)
Diagnosis; Fibrocystic disease; Mastectomy

BC0522 MY BREAST: ONE WOMAN'S CANCER STORY
Wadler, J.
New York
Apr. 20, 1992, vol. 25, n. n16, p. 48(11)
Care and treatment; Surgery

BC0523 WAS THIS OPERATION NECESSARY?
Wallis, C.
Time
Nov. 2, 1987, vol. 130, p. 78(1)
Operations, Necessary
Nancy and Ronald Reagan.

BC0524 THE ROUGH ROAD TO RECOVERY: OPTIONS FOR THERAPY HAVE MULTIPLIED, BUT MAKING THE RIGHT CHOICES CAN BE DAUNTING FOR BOTH DOCTORS AND PATIENTS
Wallis, C.
Time
Jan. 14, 1991, vol. 137, n. n2, p. 53(2)
Mammaplasty

BC0525 NEW CLUE TO HOW MEASLES SPREAD...CHEWABLE "LIFESAVER"...BREAST CANCER: MORE CHOICES
Weber, M.
Vogue
July 1985, vol. 175, p. 62(1)
Mastectomy; Antihypertensive drugs

BC0526 A COLOUR ATLAS OF OMENTAL TRANSPOSITION FOR ADVANCED BREAST CARCINOMA
White, H.
Single Surgical Procedures Series
1987, vol. 42
Surgery

BC0527 PROGRESS AGAINST BREAST CANCER

Willis, J.
FDA Consumer
May 1986, vol. 20, p. 6(6)
Mastectomy
Types of mammography. Mean exposure in roentgens. Breast self-examination.

BC0528 BREAST CANCER: DON'T SKIP THE RADIATION

Hippocrates
Sept.-Oct. 1988, vol. 2, n. n5, p. 10(1)
Radiotherapy; lumpectomy

BC0529 THE TREATMENT MAZE: WHAT TO EXPECT

Consumer Reports
Nov. 1988, vol. 53, n. n11, p. 734(2)
Treatment Maze

BC0530 CANCER IN THE CONTRALATERAL BREAST AFTER RADIOTHERAPY FOR BREAST CANCER

The New England Journal of Medicine
Mar. 19, 1992, vol. 326, p. 781-785
Breast, Contralateral

BC0531 BREAST DISEASE FOR RADIOGRAPHERS: A GUIDE

1988
Radiographers

BC0532 MEDICARE COVERAGE FOR MAMMOGRAPHY EXAMINATIONS

Committee on Ways and Means
1988, vol. III, p. 107
Mammography, Health Insurance

BC0533 REPORT TO THE MINISTER FOR HEALTH FOR WESTERN AUSTRALIA FROM THE WORKING PARTY ON SCREENING MAMMOGRAPHY

Working Party on Screening Mammography
1987, p. 73
Australia

BC0534 RAD RISKS IN YOUNG BREASTS

Science News
Nov. 11, 1989, vol. 136, n. n20, p. 311(1)
Ionizing radiation, Youth

BC0535 AVOIDING THE SCALPEL

Reader's Digest
Dec. 1990, vol. 138, n. n824, p. 150(1)
Chemotherapy; Radiotherapy

BC0536 CANCER DETECTION IN WOMEN

Committee on Labor and Human Resources
Jan. 28, 1988, vol. III, p. 250
Detection

BC0537 TREATMENT OF EARLY-STAGE BREAST CANCER

The Journal of the American Medical Association

Jan. 16, 1991, vol. 265, n. n3, p. 391(5)
Early Stage

A report is presented by a consensus panel of investigators, methodologists, specialists, and representatives of the public concerning optimal approaches to treating breast cancer. The panel report was formulated after the Consensus Development Conference on the Treatment of Early-Stage Breast Cancer, sponsored by the National Cancer Institute and the Office of Medical Applications of Research of the National Institutes of Health. It addressed mastectomy (removal of the breast and supporting tissues) compared with approaches that conserve breast tissue (removal of the tumor only, followed by radiation therapy); techniques of breast conserve breast tissue (removal of the tumor only, followed by radiation therapy); techniques of breast conservation; the role of adjuvant therapy (chemotherapy); the importance of prognostic factors; and future research directions. Studies with long-term follow-up have shown equivalent survival for patients choosing either mastectomy or breast conservation. Thus, the choice of a treatment is made based on other considerations, such as cosmetic results, psychosocial factors, or certain aspects of the patient's disease. Specific recommendations concerning breast conservation, with examination of lymph nodes in the armpit and subsequent radiation therapy, are presented. Although most patients without lymph node involvement are cured by either mastectomy or breast conservation treatment, chemotherapy further reduces recurrence by approximately one third. Considerable research is needed in this area, and all eligible women should be asked to participate. A good prognosis is associated with smaller tumors (especially those one centimeter or less in diameter); estrogen receptor-positive tumors (slightly better than receptor-negative tumors); lower grade cancers (a measure of aggressiveness); certain histologic types; and other factors. Future research should focus on eight areas: improving methods of rating cancer severity; developing better risk factor profiles; improving systemic chemotherapy regimens; learning more concerning the safety and efficacy of tamoxifen, a chemotherapeutic agent; assessing the quality of life for patients after cancer treatment; evaluating the efficacy of irradiation given as a 'booster'; and improving radiation therapy. Other articles concerning the treatment of breast cancer appear in the January 16, 1991 issue of The Journal of the American Medical Association. (Consumer Summary produced by Reliance Medical Information. Inc.)

BC0538 BREAST DISEASES: BREAST-CONSERVING THERAPY, NON-EVASIVE LESIONS, MASTOPATHY

1989, vol. XVIII, p. 548
Breast Conserving Therapy

BC0539 AVOIDING THE SCALPEL

Reader's Digest

Dec. 1990, vol. 138, n. n824, p. 150(1)
Chemotherapy; Radiotherapy

BC0540 CANCER IN THE CONTRALATERAL BREAST AFTER RADIOTHERAPY FOR BREAST CANCER

Boice, J.D. Jr.;
The New England Journal of Medicine
Mar. 19, 1992, vol. 326, n. n12, p. 781(5)
Contralateral Breast

Breast cancer patients less than 45 years-of-age who receive radiotherapy for caner in one breast may have a higher risk of developing cancer in the other breast than those who do not receive radiotherapy. A study of 655 women who developed a second breast cancer five or more years after their first cancer found that more years after their first cancer found that approximately 23 percent had received radiotherapy. Out of 1,189 breast cancer patients who did not develop a second breast cancer, 20 percent received radiotherapy. Among women under 45 years-of-age at the time of treatment, the risk of developing a second cancer was significantly higher in those who received radiotherapy than those who received other types of treatment. Women older than 45 years at the time of treatment who received radiotherapy did not have an increased risk of developing a second cancer compared to those who did not receive radiotherapy. Women with breast cancer have three times the risk of developing a second cancer compared to healthy women, regardless of whether or not they receive radiotherapy.

BC0541 VALUE OF AXILLARY DISSECTION IN ADDITION TO LUMPECTOMY AND RADIOTHERAPY IN EARLY BREAST CANCER

Cabanes, P.A.;
The Lancet
May 23, 1992, vol. 339, n. n8804, p. 1245(4)
Lymph nodes, Lumpectomy

Women with early breast cancer who have a lumpectomy may also benefit from having the lymph nodes under their arms removed, a procedure known as axillary dissection. Of 658 women with tumors less than 3 centimeters and no suspected lymph node involvement, 332 received a lumpectomy and 326 received a lumpectomy and axillary dissection. Sixty women treated with lumpectomy and axillary dissection were found to have lymph node metastases at surgery. The average follow-up for all the women was 54 months. At five years, 92.6 percent of the women who received only a lumpectomy and 96.6 percent of the women who received a lumpectomy and axillary dissection were alive. The cancer recurrence rates were similar in both groups, but cancer was less likely to recur in the lymph nodes in the women who received axillary dissection. The likelihood of preserving the breast was equally high in both groups. The women who received axillary dissection experienced no serious complications from the surgery.

BC0542 FREEDOM OF CHOICE; LESS INVASIVE SURGERY TECHNIQUES GIVE BREAST CANCER VICTIMS NEW TREATMENT OPTIONS

Dranov, P.
Saavy
July 1987, vol. 8, p. 78(2)
Radiotherapy; mastectomy; lumpectomy

BC0543 THE INFLUENCE OF DIAGNOSTIC RADIOGRAPHY ON THE INCIDENCE OF BREAST CANCER AND LEUKEMIA

Evans, J.S.; J.E.
The New England Journal of Medicine
Sept. 25, 1986, vol. 315, p. 810-815
X-rays; Health surveys

BC0544 DOES GENE HIKE RADIATION'S CANCER RISK

Ezzell, C.
Science News
Jan. 4, 1992, vol. 141, n. n1, p. 4(1)
Radiation

BC0545 EIGHT-YEAR RESULTS OF A RANDOMIZED CLINICAL TRIAL COMPARING TOTAL MASTECTOMY AND LUMPECTOMY WITH OR WITHOUT IRRADIATION IN THE TREATMENT OF BREAST CANCER

Fisher, B.; C.
The New England Journal of Medicine
Mar. 30, 1989, vol. 320, n. n13, p. 822(7)
Radiotherapy; Lymph nodes

Lumpectomy, the surgical removal of a tumor from the breast, followed by radiation therapy, was conducted in 1,843 patients suffering from Stage I or II breast cancer. Chemotherapy was used as well in those women with cancer surrounding the nodes near the breast. Lumpectomy followed by radiation therapy resulted in a five-year survival rate of 85 percent, whereas the five-year survival rate of total mastectomy was 76 percent. At follow-up eight years after initial treatments, 90 percent of the women who underwent lumpectomy followed by irradiation were free of tumors in the same breast, while only 61 percent of patients who did not receive radiation treatment remained tumor-free. In addition, 94 percent of the patients with lymph node involvement who were treated with a combination of lumpectomy, radiation, and chemotherapy had no recurrences in the breast treated. The value of radiation therapy in reducing the recurrence of tumors following lumpectomy continues to be significant. Furthermore, the data to date continue to support breast conservation (as contrasted with total mastectomy) for patients with primary breast cancer (cancer which has not moved to other sites in the body. Distribution of patients according to treatment group. (table) Life-time table analysis: percentage who remained free of breast tumor. (graph) Disease-free survival rate and cumulative incidence of events, each group. (table) Life table analysis showing rates of disease-free survival. (graph) Comparison of 5-year life-table estimates and results. (table) Comparison of mastectomy, lumpectomy, and lumpectomy with radiation therapy. (table) Lumpectomy and lumpectomy with irradiation, according to node status. (table)

BC0546 BREAST CANCER: IMPORTANCE OF ADEQUATE SURGICAL EXCISION PRIOR TO RADIOTHERAPY IN THE LOCAL CONTROL OF BREAST CANCER IN PATIENTS TREATED CONSERVATIVELY

Ghossein, N.A.
The Journal of the American Medical Association
June 24, 1992, vol. 267, n. n26, p. 3274(1)
Surgery, Radiotherapy

BC0547 THE RISK OF BREAST CANCER AFTER IRRADIATION OF THE THYMUS IN INFANCY

Hildreth, N.C.;
The New England Journal of Medicine
Nov. 9, 1989, vol 321, n. n19, p. 1281(4)
Carcinogenesis

Radiation exposure is known to cause breast cancer. Most studies have examined the effects of radiation that occur during adolescence and adulthood. One study found that women who had been exposed to radiation from the atomic bomb before age 10 have a higher incidence of breast cancer than women in the general population. Over 30 years ago an enlarged thymus gland during infancy was though to be harmful the life- threatening, and radiation was routinely used to shrink the thymus gland tissue. Later research indicated that an enlarged thymus was not abnormal and the practice of irradiating the thymus gland was stopped. To determine whether women irradiated during infancy for enlarged thymus glands had an increased risk for developing breast cancer, 1,201 women who had received such treatment were compared with 2,469 who had not. The irradiated thymus group had 22 breast cancers compared with 12 cancers within the nonirradiated group when evaluated and average of 36 years afterwards. The first cancer was diagnosed at 29 years old. It is concluded that women exposed to radiation very early in life have an increased risk for developing breast cancer many years later. Breast cancer is rare in women under 28 and it is theorized that early radiation exposure makes the breast tissue more susceptible to the tumor- promoting effects of hormones. Therefore, it is assumed that the radiation damages the breast tissue as opposed to damaging the immune system directly. Physicians are urged to act cautiously when planning early exposure to high doses of ionizing (x-ray) radiation. Risk factors for breast cancer with and without thymus radiation. (table) Radiation dose-response for breast cancer in irradiated children. (table) Estimates of breast cancer from various studies. (table)

BC0548 CANCER: FACTS VS, FEELINGS; PATIENTS ARE TREATED LIKE AIRLINE LUGGAGE: CHECKED IN, WEIGH, X-RAYED, TAGGED AND IGNORED

Kaufman, M.
Newsweek
Apr. 24, 1989, vol. 113, n. n17, p. 10(1)

BC0549 UNDERUTILIZATION OF BREAST-CONSERVING SURGERY AND RADIATION THERAPY AMONG WOMEN WITH STAGE I AND II BREAST CANCER

Lazovich, D.; E.
The Journal of the American Medical Association
Dec. 25, 1991, vol. 266, n. n24, p. 3433(6)
Lumpectomy

Traditionally, breast cancer was treat using the Halsted mastectomy, surgical removal of the breast, underlying chest muscles, and axillary contents. Recent research has indicated that among women with breast cancer in its early stages, conservative treatment involving only excision of the tumor and surrounding tissue followed by radiation therapy is preferable. Women not given radiation therapy tended to be older, to have stage II disease, or to live in an area without radiation therapy facilities. These results indicate that BCS (and in some cases radiation therapy) was underutilized as a treatment for early-stage breast cancer in this population.

BC0550 MORTALITY FROM BREAST CANCER AFTER IRRADIATION DURING FLUOROSCOPIC EXAMINATIONS IN PATIENTS BEING TREATED FOR TUBERCULOSIS

Miller, A.B.; G.R.
The New England Journal of Medicine
Nov. 9, 1989, Vol. 321, n. n19, p. 1285(5)
Mortality

High doses of radiation from X-rays and gamma rays are associated with an increased risk of breast cancer. There is some concern over the risk of low-dose radiation from mammography, the use of X-rays to visualize breast tissue and breast cancer. It is difficult to correctly assess the risk of developing cancer by studying low doses of radiation. Instead, models based on high-dose radiation effects are used to estimate the predict relationships between radiation dose and cancer development. An examination of 31,710 women was performed to evaluate the effects of this radiation on later breast cancer development. It was found that the more radiation a women was exposed to, the higher the incidence of breast cancer, particularly those irradiated between the ages of 10 to 14. The risk of breast cancer decreased sharply with increasing age in the irradiated study group. Using this model, it can be assumed that this decreased risk for breast cancer in older women supports the argument for routine mammography screening. The benefits of early detection seem to outweigh the risks of radiation-induced breast cancer.

BC0551 BREAST CANCER TRIALS: A PATIENT'S VIEWPOINT

Thronton, H.M.
The Lancet
Jan. 4, 1992, vol. 339, n. n8784, p. 44(2)
Radiotherapy

BC0552 BREAST CANCER: TWO STEPS CLOSER TO UNDERSTANDING

Wright, K.
Science
Dec. 1990, vol. 250, n. n4988, p. 1659(1)
Tumor suppressor genes

It is estimated in 1990, 44,000 patients out of the 150,000 patients diagnosed, will die from breast cancer. If patients who are at risk for breast cancer are identified, then early diagnosis can occur. With early treatment, it is felt that the deaths can be prevented. Genetic factors that may increase susceptibility to breast cancer have recently been identified. Stephen Friend and colleagues at the Massachusetts General Hospital showed that mutations in a gene called p53, which encodes a product that causes suppression of tumor development, occurs in patients with Li-Fraumeni syndrome; these patients develop breast cancer as well as other cancers. Two other reports published in the Dec 21, 1990 issue of Science, volume 250, also show hat breast cancer may develop due to a series of genetic changes. Mary Clair King and colleagues of the University of California School of Public Health found a gene that is different from the p53 gene, located on chromosome 17, which may be associated with susceptibility to breast cancer. Mark Scholnick and colleagues at the University of Utah Medical Center found that some individual s have certain genetic predispositions to the noncancerous condition known as proliferative breast disease, which may lead to breast cancer. These studies are additional evidence for the current theory that several genetic changes are necessary for the progression to cancer. These studies may lead to the development of clinical tests to identify the genetic predisposition for breast cancer, leading to earlier diagnosis and treatment. (Consumer Summary produced by Reliance Medical Information. Inc.)

BC0553 AFTER CANCER; A DRUG TO PREVENT RECURRENCE

Time

Sept. 23,1985, vol. 126, 71(1)
Tamoxifen

BC0554 RX FOR RECURRING BREAST CANCER

FDA Consumer

Mar. 1987, vol. 21, p. 3(1)
Tamoxifen

BC0555 COMBINATION ADJUVANT CHEMOTHERAPY FOR NODE-POSITIVE BREAST CANCER; INADEQUACY OF A SINGLE PERIOPERATIVE CYCLE

The New England Journal of Medicine

Sept. 15, 1988, vol. 319, n. n11, p. 677(7)
Adjuvant Therapy

Study design. Characteristics of patients. 4-year old disease-free survival percentages. Disease-free survival according to treatment group. Sites of first relapse at media follow-up. 4-year overall survival percentages.

BC0556 EFFECTS OF ADJUVANT TAMOXIFEN AND OF CYTOTOXIC THERAPY ON MORTALITY IN EARLY BREAST CANCER: AN OVERVIEW OF 61 RANDOMIZED TRIALS AMONG 28,896 WOMEN

The New England Journal of Medicine

Dec. 29, 1988, vol. 319, n. n26, p. 1681(12)
Tamoxifen; Cytotoxic Therapy

Randomized trials available for evaluation of tamoxifen and chemotherapy. Treatment groups at entry: women aged <50 years old; 50 years and older. Women aged 50 years and older at entry. Estimated survival among women in all available trials comparing regimens. Comparisons of effects of tamoxifen regimes on mortality. Comparison of clinical trials: women aged <50 years old; 50 years and older.

BC0557 PROLONGED DISEASE-FREE SURVIVAL AFTER ONE COURSE OF PERIOPERATIVE ADJUVANT CHEMOTHERAPY FOR NODE-NEGATIVE BREAST CANCER

The New England Journal of Medicine

Feb. 23, 1989, vol. 320, n. n8, p. 491(6)
Adjuvent Chemotherapy

There is a great deal of evidence that mastectomy followed by chemotherapy and endocrine therapy prolongs disease-free survival and life expectancy in patients with operable breast cancer. This has proved to be the case in patients whose breast cancer had spread into the nearby lymph nodes. The more favorable prognosis of node-negative breast cancer has made clinicians reluctant to put patients through the rigors and the expense of chemotherapy. A study was conducted to evaluate the effectiveness of administering a single cycle of combination chemotherapy, including cyclophosphamide, methotrexate, fluorouracil, and leucovorin, to patients with operable node-negative breast cancer shortly after surgery. The average four year disease-free survival rate for patients who received chemotherapy was 77 percent, compared to 73 percent for similar patients who did not receive additional therapy.

BC0558 CHEMOTHERAPY OF METASTATIC BREAST CANCER IN THE ELDERLY: THE PIEDMONT ONCOLOGY ASSOCIATION EXPERIENCE

Journal of the American Medical Association

July 1, 1992, vol. 268, p. 57-62
Clinical trials

BC0559 BREAST CANCER: PATIENTS' SURVIVAL
Washington G.A.O.
Feb. 28, 1989, p. 52
Chemotherapy

BC0560 ANTI-OESTROGENS IN ONCOLOGY: PAST, PRESENT, AND PROSPECTS
Proceedings of the International Symposium of Hormonotherapy
1985, p. 300
Anti-Oestrogens

BC0561 ESTROGEN/ANTIESTROGEN ACTION AND BREAST CANCER THERAPY
1986, vol. XXIII, P. 535
Chemotherapy

BC0562 CHEMOTHERAPY OF GYNECOLOGICAL AND BREAST CANCER
1987, vol. IX, p. 84
Chemotherapy; Gynecological Cancer

BC0563 CLINICAL PROGRESS WITH MITOXANTRONE
International Congress and Symposium Series
1986
Chemotherapy

BC0564 THE PLACE OF ENDOCRINE THERAPY IN BREAST DISEASE
International Congress and Symposium Series
1987
Endocrine Therapy

BC0565 ENDOCRINE-DEPENDENT BREAST CANCER: CRITICAL ASSESSMENT OF RECENT ADVANCES
14th International Cancer Congress
1988, p. 105
Hormone therapy

BC0566 LH-RH AGONISTS IN ONCOLOGY
1988

BC0567 ENDOCRINE THERAPY AND GROWTH REGULATION OF BREAST CANCER
1989, vol. VIII, p. 92
Endocrine Therapy; Growth Regulation

BC0568 ADJUVANT THERAPY OF PRIMARY BREAST CANCER
1989, vol. XVI, p. 296
Adjuvant Therapy

BC0569 THE ROLE OF ANTIHORMONES

1991, vol. X, p. 182
Antihormones

BC0570 ADJUVANT THERAPY OF BREAST CANCER

Cancer Treatment and Research

1992, vol. XVI, p. 464
Adjuvant Therapy

BC0571 HORMONE REPLACEMENT THERAPY AND BREAST CANCER RISK

1992, vol. XII, p. 321
Hormone Replacement Therapy

BC0572 ADJUVANT THERAPY OF BREAST CANCER IV

1993
Adjuvant Therapy

BC0573 AVOIDING THE SCALPEL

Reader's Digest

Mar. 1991, vol. 138, n. n827, p. 96(1)
Chemotherapy; Radiotherapy

BC0574 ADJUVANT SYSTEMATIC THERAPY FOR EARLY BREAST CANCER

The Lancet

Jan. 4, 1992, vol. 339, n. n8784, p. 27(1)
Adjuvant Systematic Therapy
A review of 133 trials of adjuvant therapy in early breast cancer involving 75,000 women showed this treatment can improve 10-year survival. Although the numbers are small -- only a dozen additional survivors for every 100 women with stage II disease and a dozen for every 200 women with stage I -- this could result in 100,000 additional survivors for every 1 million women treated.

BC0575 LONG-TERM BREAST CANCER BENEFIT SEEN

Facts on File

Jan. 9, 1992, vol. 52, n. n2668, p. 12(1)
Chemotherapy; Hormone therapy

BC0576 DRAMATIC RESULTS FROM DRUG THERAPY

USA Today

Feb. 1992, vol. 120, n. n2561, p. 5(1)
Drug Therapy

BC0577 TREATMENT OF EARLY-STAGE BREAST CANCER

The Journal of the American Medical Association

Jan. 16, 1991, vol. 265, n. n3, p. 391(5)

A report is presented by a consensus panel of investigators, methodologists, specialists, and representatives of the public concerning optimal approaches to treating breast cancer. The panel report was formulated after the Consensus Development Conference on the Treatment of Early-Stage Breast Cancer, sponsored by the National Cancer Institute and the Office of Medical Applications of Research of the National Institutes of Health. It addressed mastectomy (removal of the breast and supporting tissues) compared with approaches that conserve breast tissue (removal of the tumor only, followed by radiation therapy); techniques of breast conserve breast tissue (removal of the tumor only, followed by radiation therapy); techniques of breast conservation; the role of adjuvant therapy (chemotherapy); the importance of prognostic factors; and future research directions. Studies with long-term follow-up have shown equivalent survival for patients choosing either mastectomy or breast conservation. Thus, the choice of a treatment is made based on other considerations, such as cosmetic results, psychosocial factors, or certain aspects of the patient's disease. Specific recommendations concerning breast conservation, with examination of lymph nodes in the armpit and subsequent radiation therapy, are presented. Although most patients without lymph node involvement are cured by either mastectomy or breast conservation treatment, chemotherapy further reduces recurrence by approximately one third. Considerable research is needed in this area, and all eligible women should be asked to participate. A good prognosis is associated with smaller tumors (especially those one centimeter or less in diameter); estrogen receptor-positive tumors (slightly better than receptor-negative tumors); lower grade cancers (a measure of aggressiveness); certain histologic types; and other factors. Future research should focus on eight areas: improving methods of rating cancer severity; developing better risk factor profiles; improving systemic chemotherapy regimens; learning more concerning the safety and efficacy of tamoxifen, a chemotherapeutic agent; assessing the quality of life for patients after cancer treatment; evaluating the efficacy of irradiation given as a 'booster'; and improving radiation therapy. Other articles concerning the treatment of breast cancer appear in the January 16, 1991 issue of The Journal of the American Medical Association. (Consumer Summary produced by Reliance Medical Information. Inc.)

BC0578 COMBINE TREATMENTS FOR BEST RESULTS

USA Today

Oct. 1991, vol. 120, n. n2557, p. 4(1)
Mastectomy; Radiotherapy; Chemotherapy

BC0579 AVOIDING THE SCALPEL

Reader's Digest

Dec. 1990, vol. 138, n. n824, p. 150(1)
Chemotherapy; Radiotherapy

BC0580 SYSTEMATIC TREATMENT OF EARLY BREAST CANCER BY HORMONAL, CYTOTOXIC, OR IMMUNE THERAPY: 133 RANDOMIZED TRIALS INVOLVING 31,000 RECURRENCES AND 24,000 DEATHS AMONG 75,000 WOMEN

The Lancet

Jan. 4, 1992, vol. 339, n. n8784, p. 1(15)
Adjuvant treatment
Hormonal treatment of early breast cancer may reduce the rate of disease recurrence and prolong survival. Data on 133 worldwide trails of adjuvant treatment of breast cancer begun before 1985 and involving 75,000 women were reviewed. Of those women, 30,000 were participating in trials of tamoxifen, an anti-estrogen that blocks the stimulation of the tumor by estrogen. After 10 years, 58.8 percent of the women taking tamoxifen were alive compared to 52.6 percent of the control group, that is, women were not taking tamoxifen. Fifty-one percent of the women in the tamoxifen group were disease-free at 10 years compared to 44.7 percent of the control group. The data from 3,000 women enrolled in ovarian ablation trials were also reviewed. Ovarian ablation involves removing the ovaries -- which produce estrogen -- or inactivating them with radiation or drugs. In women under 50, 52.9 percent in the ovarian ablation group were alive after 15 years compared to 42.3 percent in the control group.

BC0581 TARGETING THE SUPPLY LINES

Allison, M.
Harvard Health Letter

May 1991, vol. 16, n. n7, p. 2(3)
Tumors

BC0582 THE TAKE-CHARGE PATIENT

Atkins, A.
Ladies' Home Journal

Nov. 1990, vol. 107, n. n11, p. 163(6)
Menopause; Hysterectomy; Mastectomy
Hysterectomy and its possible alternatives. (table) Hormone-replacement therapy. (table) Treating breast cancer. (table)

BC0583 UNDER THE SHADOW OF CANCER

Bergholz, E.
The New York Times Magazine

Dec. 11, 1988, vol. 138, p. 73
Chemotherapy

BC0584 DIAGNOSIS: MALIGNANT

Bolick, N.O.
Boston

July 1985, vol. 77, p. 104(6)
Chemotherapy

BC0585 ESTROGEN REPLACEMENT THERAPY AFTER BREAST CANCER

Burns, E.E. and
The Journal of the American Medical Association

Jan. 22, 1992, vol. 267, n. n4, p. 568(1)
Estrogen Repalcement Therapy

BC0586 WARDING OFF BREAST CANCER; BRITISH TRY TAMOXIFEN FOR HIGH-RISK WOMEN

Carpi, J.
American Health

Oct. 1990, vol. 9, n. n8, p. 10(1)
Britian, Tamoxifen

BC0587 CHEMOTHERAPY OF METASTATIC BREAST CANCER IN THE ELDERLY: THE PIEDMONT ONCOLOGY ASSOCIATION EXPERIENCE

Christman, K.;

The Journal of the American Medical Association

July 1, 1992, vol. 268, n. n1, p. 57(6)

Chemotherapy, Metastatic Cancer

Women over 70 years old who have advanced breast cancer may respond to chemotherapy as well as younger women. Many elderly women are excluded from chemotherapy trails or are given a lower dose because they are thought to have an increased risk of side effects. Of 161 women with advanced breast cancer selected from five different chemotherapy trails, 70 were over 70 years old and 91 were younger. There were no differences in response, progression of disease or survival between the older women and the younger women. The older women were more likely to develop neutropenia, which is a drop in the level of a type of white blood cell. Neutropenia was the cause of death in one elderly woman. Elderly women with advanced breast caner could be given colony stimulating factors, which are naturally-occurring substances in the body that boost the production of white blood cells.

BC0588 IMPROVING THE QUALITY OF LIFE DURING CHEMOTHERAPY FOR ADVANCED BREAST CANCER; A COMPARISON OF INTERMITTENT AND CONTINUOUS TREATMENT STRATEGIES

Coates, A.; V.

The New England Journal of Medicine

Dec. 10, 1987, vol. 317, n. n24, p. 1490(6)

Chemotherapy

Patient characteristics. Treatment plan. Best overall treatment response. Time to disease progression. Survival. Toxic effects and cell counts. Changes in quality-of-life scores.

BC0589 TAMOXIFEN-PANACEA OR PANDORA'S BOX?

Davidson, N.E.

The New England Journal of Medicine

Mar. 26, 1992, vol. 326, n. n13, p. 885(2)

Drug therapy

The anti-estrogen drug tamoxifen can improve survival and decrease cancer recurrence in women with breast cancer, but the drug also has side effects. Women over 50 years-old who are treated with tamoxifen may have fewer cancer recurrences, and fewer occurrences of cancer in the other breast. In a study of postmenopausal women with breast cancer, tamoxifen preserved bone density in the spine, but not in the forearm. Tamoxifen may only effect a certain type of bone. The spine contains this type of bone, but the forearm does not. Patients treated tamoxifen have reduced cholesterol levels, and decreased risk of death from cardiovascular disease. Premenopausal women treated with tamoxifen can remain fertile, but the effects of tamoxifen on fetuses is unknown. The drug may cause hormonal changes, blood clots, eye abnormalities and second cancers. A proposed study will examine whether tamoxifen can prevent breast cancer in 16,000 healthy women with a high risk of breast cancer.

BC0590 BREAST CANCER THERAPY: EXERCISING ALL OUR OPTIONS
DeVita, V.T. Jr.
The New England Journal of Medicine
Feb. 23, 1989, vol. 320, n n8 p. 527(3)
Chemotherapy

Each year in the US about 70,000 women develop axillary node-negative breast cancer. Chemotherapy is used as an adjuvant to mastectomy and has been tested as a means of reducing the likelihood of cancer recurrence. Other important features of adjuvant therapy are the minimal toxicity of some of the chemotherapeutic programs, and the complementary use of tamoxifen with radiotherapy. More intensive chemotherapy may result in increased toxicity to the patient, but this should be offset by the convenience of a shorter duration of treatment, especially if results are enhanced. Seventy percent of node-negative breast cancer patients would not have a recurrence if they received no additional treatment after mastectomy, but currently these patients can not be identified. Patients can now be offered mastectomy with improved cosmetic results and short term chemotherapy with markedly reduced toxicity as a means of preventing recurrence and prolong life. The findings indicate that women with newly diagnosed localized invasive breast cancer can and should be offered some form of systemic treatment either in or outside the confines of a clinical trial.

BC0591 THE WISEST DECISION I EVER MADE
Eaton, E. and J.
Good Housekeeping
July 1987, vol. 205, p. 48(4)
Pregnancy

BC0592 DRUGS GIVE SLIGHT EDGE IN BREAST CANCER
Fackelmann, K.A.
Science News
Mar. 4, 1989, vol. 135 n. n9, p. 135(1)
Chemotherapy

BC0593 THE ADJUVANT ADVANTAGE: BREAST CANCER THERAPIES PROMISE A LONGER LIFE
Fackelmann, K.A.
Science News
Feb. 22, 1992, vol. 141, n. n8, p. 124(2)
Yew; Taxol

BC0594 A RANDOMIZED CLINICAL TRIAL EVALUATING SEQUENTIAL METHOTREXATE AND FLUOROURACIL IN THE TREATMENT OF PATIENTS WITH NODE-NEGATIVE BREAST CANCER WHO HAVE ESTROGEN-RECEPTOR-NEGATIVE TUMORS
Fisher, B.; C.
The New England Journal of Medicine
Feb. 23, 1989, vol. 320, n. n8, p. 473(6)
Methotrexate; Fluorouracil

Methotrexate and fluorouracil were administered to women following removal of breast tumors as a means of preventing recurrence of cancer in patients whose tumor cells did not have estrogen receptors and whose cancer had not spread to lymph nodes. Research findings indicate that these chemotherapeutic agents prolong disease-free survival in all patients who receive them with moderate and easily controlled toxic side-effects. It was necessary for the breast tumors to be large enough so that the estrogen-receptor concentration could be measured by conventional methods.

BC0595 A RANDOMIZED CLINICAL TRIAL EVALUATING TAMOXIFEN IN THE TREATMENT OF PATIENTS WITH NODE-NEGATIVE BREAST CANCER WHO HAVE ESTROGEN-RECEPTOR-POSITIVE TUMORS

Fisher, B.; J.
The New England Journal of Medicine
Feb. 23, 1989, vol. 320, n. n8, p. 479(6)
Tamoxifen

A randomized double-blind study of tamoxifen in post-operative therapy among 2644 women who had a malignant breast tumor removed id presented. All of the patients in this study had node-negative cancer and estrogen-receptor-positive tumors. results of the study indicate that tamoxifen prolongs the disease-free survival of women who have estrogen-receptor-positive breast tumors and has fewer toxic side effects. The effect of tamoxifen may be related more to suppression of existing tumor growth rather than the prevention of the new tumor growth. The degree of benefit achieved with tamoxifen is not sufficient to eliminate the need for future trials to evaluate potentially more effective therapies. Randomization, eligibility and follow-up in population considered for study. Characteristics of patients with follow-up data. Disease-free survival according to treatment and age group. Sites of treatment failure. Reasons reported for stopping treatment. Incidence of common symptoms occurring after therapy, according to age.

BC0596 BEATING BREAST CANCER

Gorman, C.
Time
Jan. 13, 1992, vol. 139, n. n2, p. 50(1)

BC0597 BREAST CANCER THERAPY-THE PRICE OF SUCCESS

Henderson, I.C.
The New England Journal of Medicine
June 25, 1992, vol. 326, n. n26, p. 1774(2)
Leukemia; Chemotherapy

Over half of all women diagnosed with breast cancer will be cured. A recent report found that the risk of developing leukemia is higher in women with breast cancer who have been treated with drugs that are commonly used in chemotherapy. However, the risk is low, and must be balanced against the reduction in mortality from breast cancer in patients receiving chemotherapy. Another report discussed the characteristics of tumors that would determine the patient's prognosis. Tumor size and the presence of metastases to the lymph nodes appear to be the best predictors of survival. Many patients may have a combination of good and bad prognostic factors, and physicians may prefer to treat such patients. Prognostic factors can not replace a doctor's clinical judgment, or his consultation with his colleagues and the patient concerning the most appropriate treatment.

BC0598 EFFICACY AND COST EFFECTIVENESS OF ADJUVANT CHEMOTHERAPY IN WOMEN WITH NODE-NEGATIVE BREAST CANCER

Hillner, B.E.; T.J.
The New England Journal of Medicine
Jan. 17, 1991, vol. 324, n. n3, p. 160(9)
Adjuvant Chemotherapy

The 1988 Clinical Alert issued by the National Caner Institute indicated that chemotherapy had meaningful effects on the development of disease in women with node-negative breast cancer. This has been widely interpreted as suggesting that chemotherapy should be used more extensively. Since the majority of women with breast cancer whose disease has not yet spread to the lymph nodes of the armpit will achieve long-term survival without chemotherapy, it is important to examine both the costs and benefits of chemotherapy for these patients. It is clear that the use of chemotherapy for node-negative breast cancer patients would result in the needless treatment of many women. In addition, the aggregate yearly cost of this additional treatment would be roughly $338 million. The authors investigated the potential benefits of expanding the use of chemotherapy by developing a Markov model of node-negative breast cancer. (Markov models are probabilistic models; named for the Russian mathematician Markov, they are generally used in cases where a system can progress through possible states and the probability of moving into a new state is determined only by the state the system is in.) The model evaluated the cost-effectiveness of chemotherapy for 45- and 60-year-old woman under varying sets of assumptions. The investigators found that for the standard assumptions, the 60-year-old woman gained about four months of quality life at a cost of $18,800 per year while the 45-year-old woman gained 5.1 months at a cost of $15,400 per year. Unfortunately, little is known about the differences between women with node-negative cancer and high risk of recurrence and those with low risk of recurrence. If it turns out that chemotherapy is not equally effective in both groups, then the chemotherapy is less effective. Furthermore, improved disease-free survival resulting from chemotherapy may not result in improved overall survival, and this, too, may affect the expectations. The authors suggest that the uncertainty is too great for many women to choose chemotherapy. However, the authors hope that it might be possible to identify a subset of high-risk patients who might gain proportionately more from chemotherapy. Unfortunately, can actually be accomplished with the knowledge at hand. (Consumer Summary produced by Reliance Medical Information. Inc.) Abbreviated version of the markov model used in this study. (chart) Health states in the study model and their incremental values. (table) Alternative models of the duration of survival. (graph) Probability of recurrence, complications, chemotherapy, and death. (table) Base-line analyses in two cohorts. (table) Sensitivity analyses in the 45-year-old cohorts. (graph) Structural sensitivity analyses. (graph)

BC0599 THE BIG SWITCH IN BREAST CANCER TREATMENT

Holland, L.
Good Housekeeping
Sept. 1988, vol. 207, n. n3, p. 273(2)
Chemotherapy; hormone therapy

Odds of getting and surviving breast cancer. American Cancer Society guidelines for early detection.

BC0600 WONDER DRUG? TEST MAY GIVE ANSWER ON ICI'S TAMOXIFEN

Kent, W.

Barron's National Business and Financial Weekly

Sept. 30, 1991, vol. 71, n. n39, p. 18(2)
Pharmaceutical industry

BC0601 BREAST CANCER CONSENSUS

Kolata, G.

Science

Sept. 27, 1985, vol. 229, p. 1378(1)
Chemotherapy; Hormone therapy; Drug therapy

BC0602 THE THROMBOGENIC EFFECT OF ANTICANCER DRUG THERAPY IN WOMEN WITH STAGE II BREAST CANCER

Levine, M.N.; M.

The New England Journal of Medicine

Feb. 18, 1988, vol. 318, n. n7, p. 404(4)
Antineoplastic agents; pulmonary embolism; chemotherapy Characteristics of patient groups.

BC0603 THE MOST VERSATILE DRUG TODAY?

Lippert, J.

Ladies' Home Journal

Sept. 1992, vol. 109, n. n9, p. 144(1)
Osteogenesis; Menopause

BC0604 EFFECTS OF TAMOXIFEN ON BONE MINERAL DENSITY IN POSTMENOPAUSAL WOMEN WITH BREAST CANCER

Love, R.R.; Mazess; R.B. Barden; H.S.

The New England Journal of Medicine

Mar. 26, 1992, vol. 326, n. n13, p. 852(5)
Tamoxifen, Bone Mineral Density
Postmenopausal women with breast cancer who are treated with tamoxifen may not suffer from the decrease in bone density that usually occurs after menopause. Tamoxifen is a drug given to women with breast cancer after primary chemotherapy for five to 10-year periods. Out of 140 postmenopausal women with breast cancer, 70 received 10 milligrams (mg) of oral tamoxifen twice a day, and 70 were treated with placebo, an inactive substance. Bone mineral density of the spine and forearm were evaluated at different times over a two-year period. Spinal bone density decreased in both groups. T

BC0605 EFFICACY OF ADJUVANT CHEMOTHERAPY IN HIGH-RISK NODE-NEGATIVE BREAST CANCER: AN INTERGROUP STUDY

Mansour, E.G; Gray; A.H. Shatila, C.K.

The New England Journal of Medicine

Feb. 23, 1989, vol. 320, n. n8, p. 485(6)
Cyclophosphamide; methotrexate; fluorouracil; prednisone
Adjuvant therapy is required in the treatment of primary breast cancer when the cancer has spread to lymph nodes near the breast. High cancer recurrence and death rates in women whose breast cancer is node-negative led researchers to assess the effectiveness of adjuvant chemotherapy for these patients. After radical or modified mastectomy, patients were observed or were administered short-term intensive chemotherapy, using cyclophoshamide, methrotrexate, fluorouracil, and prednisone. These node-negative patients had either a tumor of any size without estrogen receptors or a tumor greater than or equal to three centimeters with estrogen receptors. The disease-free survival rate among patients treated with adjuvant chemotherapy was 84 percent and 69 percent for the patients who were observed. Severe toxicity occurred in 33 percent of the treated patients.

BC0606 ADJUVANT OF NODE-NEGATIVE BREAST CANCER

McGuire, W.L.
The New England Journal of Medicine
Feb. 23, 1989, vol. 320, n. n8, p. 525(3)
Adjuvant Therapy

BC0607 NEW EVIDENCE MAY EXPAND INDICATIONS FOR CHEMOTHERAPY IN BREAST CANCER

Merz, B.
The Journal of the American Medical Association
Sept. 1, 1989, vol. 262, n. n9, p. 1153(1)
Mastectomy

A study has found that mortality among women being treated for breast cancer by surgical tumor resection combined with chemotherapy is lower than the mortality of women treated with a combination of radiation therapy and mastectomy. The use of chemotherapy drug tamoxifen reduced the change of death by 20 percent per year in breast cancer patients women over 50 years of age and by 25 percent in younger women. Chemotherapy treatment which includes a combination of drugs is more effective than the use of a single chemotherapeutic agent. Another study followed 97 candidates for modified radical mastectomy. Chemotherapy reduced the tumors sufficiently in 87 percent of the patients to allow a conservative resection. Chemotherapy should not be the only treatment choice for women with breast cancer, but there is good evidence for more widespread use of it.

BC0608 INTERRUPTED VERSUS CONTINUOUS CHEMOTHERAPY IN PATIENTS WITH METASTATIC BREAST CANCER

Muss, H.B.; L.D.
The New England Journal of Medicine
Nov. 7, 1991, vol. 325, n. n19, p. 1342(7)
Chemotherapy

In breast cancer, as in most cancers, the most serious complication involves the ability of the cancer cells to spread through the body and grow as secondary cancers in organs distant from the primary cancer. Metastatic breast cancer is essentially incurable, and once breast cancer has reached this stage, chemotherapeutic treatment is administered for the palliation of symptoms, rather than with hopes of increasing survival. It is not certain, however, what the optimal type of chemotherapeutic treatment might be under these circumstances. Many patients with advanced breast cancer are given chemotherapy continuously, but research on some other forms of cancer has indicated that interrupted chemotherapy may be equally effective for relieving symptoms. Since chemotherapeutic treatment itself has serious side effects, it is important to determine if the patient is, indeed, achieving some advantage from such an unpleasant regime. This question was examined in the course of treating 250 women with metastatic breast cancer.

BC0609 TANTALIZING CLUES TO A LEGACY: RESEARCH INTO THE GENETIC FACTORS IS RAISING HOPES OF BETTER SCREENING AND TREATMENT

Nash, J.M.
Time
Jan. 14, 1991, vol. 137, n. n2, p. 55(1)

BC0610 TAMOXIFEN QUANDARY: PROMISING CANCER DRUG MAY HIDE A TROUBLING DARK SIDE
Raloff, J.
Science News
Apr. 25, 1992, vol. 141, n. n17, p. 266(4)

BC0611 TAMOXIFEN TRIAL BEGINS AMID NEW CONCERNS
Ratloff, J.
Science News
May 9, 1992, vol. 141, n. n19, p. 309(1)
Tamoxifen

BC0612 BREAST CANCER: WHEN CHEMOTHERAPY WORKS
Rennie, S.
Ms.
Nov. 1987, vol. 16, p. 70(5)
Chemotherapy
Postsurgery prognosis.

BC0613 BREAST CANCER: WHEN CHEMOTHERAPY WORKS
Rennie, S.
Ms.
Nov. 1987, vol. 16, p. 70-74
Chemotherapy

BC0614 TAMOXIFEN QUANDARY
Roloff, J.
Science News
Apr. 25, 1992, vol. 141, p. 266-269
Pharmaceutical research; chemotherapy; risk; medical care

BC0615 CHEMOTHERAPY AND THE BREAST CANCER PATIENT
Saline, C.
Philadelphia Magazine
Mar. 1989, vol. 80, n. n3, p. 41(3)
Chemotherapy

BC0616 CHEMOTHERAPY AND THE BREAST CANCER PATIENT
Saline, C.
Philadelphia Magazine
Mar. 1989, vol. 80, n. n3, p. 41(3)
Chemotherapy

BC0617 GOOD FOR YEW
Sangiorgio, M.; G.
Prevention
Feb. 1992, vol. 44, n. n2, p. 18(1)
Taxol; Ovarian cancer

BC0618 WINNING THE CHEMO BATTLE
Slaton-Mitchell,
1988, p. 221
Chemiotherapy

BC0619 PROTECTIVE EFFECT OF THE BISPIPERAZINEDIONE ICRF-187 AGAINST DOXORUBICIN-INDUCED CARDIAC TOXICITY IN WOMEN WITH ADVANCED BREAST CANCER

Speyer, J.L. Green, M.D. Kramer, E. Rey, M. et al.
The New England Journal of Medicine
Sept. 22, 1988, vol. 319, n12, p. 745(8)
Women; Bispiperazinedione
Characteristics of the study groups. Cycles of treatment received and dose of doxorubicin. Percent of patients remaining free of disease progression. Noncardiac toxic effects. Mean fall from base line in the resting LVEF.

BC0620 PREVENTING BREAST CANCER: IS THIS DRUG TOO GOOD TO BE TRUE?

Wartik, N.
American Health
Sept. 1991, vol. 10, n. n7, p. 9(2)
Barring cancer: tactics to reduce your risk for specific cancers. (table)

BC0621 TAMOXIFEN AND BREAST CANCER: NEW CHOICES

Weber, M.
Vogue
Jan. 1989, vol. 179, n. n1, p. 114(1)
Tamoxifen

BC0622 CANCER

Best Buys and Discount Prices
Apr. 1986, vol 408, P. 353(16)
Chemotherapy; Radiation; Immunotherapy; Hyperthermia
The seven warning signals of cancer. How cancer spreads. Malignant and benign tumors. Breast self-examination.

BC0623 ADJUVANT THERAPY FOR BREAST CANCER: NCI RECOMMENDATIONS RAISE SERIOUS CONCERNS; HERE'S OUR PERSPECTIVE

Mayo Clinic Health Letter
Sept. 1988, vol. 6, n. n9, p. 8(1)
Adjuvant Therapy

BC0624 ENDOCRINE THERAPIES IN BREAST AND PROSTATE CANCER

1988, vol. XII, p. 161
Endorine Therapy; Prostate Cancers

BC0625 ADDITIONAL USE FOR TAMOXIFEN

FDA Consumer
Sept. 1990, Vol. 24, n. n7, p. 2(2)
Tamoxifen

BC0626 PRIMARY CHEMOTHERAPY TO AVOID MASTECTOMY IN TUMORS WITH DIAMETERS OF THREE CENTIMETERS OF MORE

The Journal of the American Medical Association

Feb. 20, 1991, vol. 265, n. n7, p. 861(1)
Adjuvant Chemotherapy

BC0627 SYSTEMATIC TREATMENT OF EARLY BREAST CANCER BY HORMONAL, CYTOTOXIC, OR IMMUNE THERAPY: 133 RANDOMIZED TRIALS INVOLVING 31,000 RECURRENCES AND 24,000 DEATHS AMONG 75,000 WOMEN

The Lancet

Jan. 4, 1992, vol. 339, n. n8784, p. 1(15)
Adjuvant treatment

Hormonal treatment of early breast cancer may reduce the rate of disease recurrence and prolong survival. Data on 133 worldwide trails of adjuvant treatment of breast cancer begun before 1985 and involving 75,000 women were reviewed. Of those women, 30,000 were participating in trials of tamoxifen, an anti-estrogen that blocks the stimulation of the tumor by estrogen. After 10 years, 58.8 percent of the women taking tamoxifen were alive compared to 52.6 percent of the control group, that is, women were not taking tamoxifen. Fifty-one percent of the women in the tamoxifen group were disease-free at 10 years compared to 44.7 percent of the control group. The data from 3,000 women enrolled in ovarian ablation trials were also reviewed. Ovarian ablation involves removing the ovaries -- which produce estrogen -- or inactivating them with radiation or drugs. In women under 50, 52.9 percent in the ovarian ablation group were alive after 15 years compared to 42.3 percent in the control group.

BC0628 BREAST CANCER TREATMENTS

Cimons, M.; A.
50 Plus

Oct. 1990, vol. 30, n. n10, p. 44(3)
Lumpectomy; Mastectomy; Mammography

BC0629 ANTICANCER DRUGS: IN VIVO LA DIFFERENCE

Decker, C.
Science News

Mar. 24, 1990, vol. 137, n. n12, p. 183(1)
Antineoplastic agents; Chemotherapy

BC0630 ADJUVANT THERAPY FOR BREAST CANCER

Henderson, I.C.
The New England Journal of Medicine

Feb. 18, 1988, vol. 318, n. n7, p. 443(2)
Antineoplastic agents

BC0631 EFFICACY AND COST-EFFECTIVENESS OF AUTOLOGOUS BONE MARROW TRANSPLANTATION IN METASTATIC BREAST CANCER: ESTIMATES USING DECISION ANALYSIS WHILE AWAITING CLINICAL TRIAL RESULTS

Hillner, B.E. ; T.J.
The Journal of the American Medical Association
Apr. 15, 1992, vol. 267, n. n15, p. 2055(7)
Care and treatment; Autografts

Patients with metastatic breast cancer may benefit from autologous bone marrow transplantation (ABMT), but this treatment may be too expensive for widespread use. Patients who receive ABMT are infused with their own bone marrow to strengthen their immune system after chemotherapy. A mathematical model was used to estimate the survival time and cost of treatment for a hypothetical group of 45-year-old women with metastatic breast cancer who were treated with high dose chemotherapy followed by ABMT, or with standard chemotherapy. One year after starting treatment, 36.1 percent of the patients who received intensive chemotherapy followed by ABMT were in complete remission, compared to 8.2 percent of the patients treated with standard chemotherapy. Five years after treatment, average survival time for patients who received intensive chemotherapy followed by ABMT was 27.4 months, and average survival time for patients who received standard chemotherapy was 21.4 months. The cost of ABMT was $115,800 per year of life saved.

BC0632 GERM LINE P53 MUTATIONS IN A FAMILIAL SYNDROME OF BREAST CANCER, SARCOMAS, AND OTHER NEOPLASMS

Malkin, D.; Li; F.P. L.C. Strong; J.F.Fraumen
Science
Nov. 30, 1990, vol. 250, n. n4985, p. 1233(6)
Sarcomas; Germ Line P53

Individuals with Li-Fraumeni syndrome, a rare genetic disorder, have a high risk of developing several malignant tumors at an unusually early age, with a consequent high death rate. The types of tumors that develop in individuals with Li-Fraumeni syndrome include cancers of the breast, soft tissues, brain, bone, adrenal gland, and blood cells. The genetic defect of Li-Fraumeni syndrome has been located in a gene which encodes a protein known as p53. This gene is known as a tumor suppressor gene. Mutations (genetic changes) in p53 can cause uncontrolled cell growth or cancer. Mutations in p53 were identified in various types of tumors from members of five families with Li-Fraumeni syndrome. The p53 protein was not produced in individuals with the mutated gene. The identification of the gene that causes the tumor development in patients with Li-Fraumeni syndrome will allow the study of the effect of the inactivation of this gene on cancer development.

BC0633 GENETIC DEFECT IDENTIFIED IN RARE CANCER SYNDROME

Marx, J.
Science
Nov. 30, 1990, vol. 250, n. n4985, p. 1209(1)
Tumor suppressor genes; Li-Fraumeni syndrome
There are approximately 100 families in the world known to have Li-Fraumeni syndrome, a rare genetic disorder, in which individuals have a high risk of developing several types of malignant tumor, especially breast cancer, at an unusually early age and with a consequent high death rate. The Li-Fraumeni syndrome is evidence that cancer can be inherited. The genetic defect of Li-Fraumeni syndrome has been identified by Stephen Friend and colleagues at Massachusetts General Hospital Cancer Center in Boston. The defect is in a gene which encodes a protein known as p53. The gene is a tumor suppressor gene, in which a mutation, or genetic defect will allow identification of members of families with Li-Fraumeni syndrome who carry the defect gene and are at high risk of developing cancer. These individual can be monitored so that any cancer can be detected early, when it is most easily treated.

BC0634 IMMUNOCYTOCHEMISTRY FOR STEROID RECEPTORS

Pertschuk, L.P.
1990, p. 210
Immunodiagnosis

BC0635 BREAST CANCER AND SENSE OF SMELL

Science News
Sept. 7, 1985, vol. 128, p. 153(1)
Smell

BC0636 BREAST CANCER IN MEN

The Harvard Medical School Health Letter
Sept. 1986, vol. 11, p. 8(1)
Men

BC0637 ESTROGENS EXONERATED IN BREAST CANCER

Science News
Jan. 24, 1987, vol. 131, p. 57(1)
Carcinogenesis

BC0638 BREAST CANCER: NEU CLUE

Scientific American
Mar. 1987, vol. 256, p. 71(2)
Oncogenes

BC0639 ONCOLOGY

The Journal of the American Medical Association
Oct. 23, 1987, vol. 258, n. n16, p. 2261(3)

BC0640 PREMATURE MORTALITY DUE TO BREAST CANCER- UNITED STATES, 1984

JAMA: The Journal of the American Medical Association
Dec. 11, 1987, vol. 258, n. n22, p. 3229(3)
United States
Projected YPLL rates. Estimated years of potential life lost before age 65.

BC0641 CANCER

Best Buys and Discount Prices
Jan. 30, 1989, vol. 497, p. 550(19)
Bladder cancer; bones--cancer; cervical cancer; colorectal cancer; leukemia; liver cancer; lung cancer; lymphomas; ovarian cancer;

BC0642 ASSURING THE QUALITY OF HEALTH CARE FOR OLDER PERSONS: AN EXPERT PANEL'S PRIORITIES
Journal of the American Medical Association
Oct. 9, 1987, vol. 258, p. 1905-1908
Senior Citizens

BC0643 CANCER: SPECIAL REPORTS
Discover
Mar. 1986, vol. 7, p. 36-41, 44-47, 50-51, 54-55, 58, 60, 62-66
Cancer research; Lung cancer

BC0644 FAILING HEALTH: A WASTEFUL SYSTEM THAT DOESN'T WORK
Progressive
Oct. 1990, vol. 54, p. 14-29
Medical economics; Health insurance; Costs/medicine--[u.s.]--costs; Occupational health and safety; Medical screening; Research

BC0645 HOSPITAL VARIABLES ASSOCIATED WITH QUALITY OF CARE FOR BREAST CANCER PATIENTS
Journal of the American Medical Association
Dec, 25, 1991, vol. 266, p. 3429-3432
Hospital Care

BC0646 UNDERGROUND MEDICINE
U.S. News and World Report
May 11, 1992, vol. 112, p. 62-71
Pharmaceutical research; clinical traits; drug policy

BC0647 BREAST AND CERVICAL CANCER MORTALITY PREVENTION ACT OF 1990
U.S. Congress. House. Committee on Energy and Commerce
1990, p. 21
Cervical Cancer

BC0648 WOMEN'S HEALTH
Washington G.P.O.
Apr. 23-25, 1990, p. 262
Cervical cancer

BC0649 BREAST CANCER DETECTION: THE NEED FOR A FEDERAL RESPONSE
Washington G.P.O.
Oct. 23, 1985, p. 169
Detection

BC0650 BREAST CANCER: RACE FOR THE CURE
Washington G.P.O.
May 16, 1990, p. 125
Cures

BC0651 BREAST CANCER ON LONG ISLAND: AN AVOIDABLE TRAGEDY?
Washington G.P.O.
Sept. 13, 1991, p. 172
Long Island

BC0652 BREAST AND CERVICAL CANCER MORTALITY PREVENTION ACT OF 1990
Washington G.P.O.
1990, p. 32
Preventive medicine; women's health services

BC0653 WHY ARE WE LOSING THE WAR ON BREAST CANCER?
Washington G.P.O.
June 20, 1991, p. 70

BC0654 WHY CONSERVATIVES DON'T TALK ABOUT AMERICA'S HEALTH SYSTEM
Washington, Democratic Study Group
1991, p. 66
Medical economics; health insurance; heart diseases

BC0655 BREAST DISEASE
Clinical Surgery International
1986, vol. 10

BC0656 PATHOLOGIE NEOPLASTISCHER UND ENDOKRIN BEDINGTER ERKRNKUNGEN DER MAMMA
Deutsche Gesellschaft fur Pathologie
1985, p. 743

BC0657 BREAST CANCER: ORIGINS, DETECTION, AND TREATMENT
Proceedings of the International Breast Cancer Research Conference
1986, vol. XVII, p. 343

BC0658 ENDOCRINOLOGY OF THE BREAST: BASIC AND CLINICAL ASPECTS
Proceedings of the International Congress on Endocrinology of the
1986, vol. XVI, p. 640
Endocrinolgy

BC0659 PATHOLOGY OF NEOPLASTIC AND ENDOCRINE INDUCED DISEASES OF THE BREAST
69th Meeting of the German Society of Pathology
1986, vol. X, p. 484
Pathology

BC0660 GENETIC EPIDEMIOLOGY: APPLICATIONS AND COMPARISONS OF METHODS
Proceedings of Genetic Analysis Workshop IV
1987, vol. XIX, p. 406
Genetic Epidemiology

BC0661 NEW FRONTIERS IN MAMMARY PATHOLOGY
Third Symposium of the International Society against Breast Cancer
1986, vol. X, p. 452
Mammary Pathology

BC0662 CANCER GENETICS IN WOMEN
1987 vol. 2
Genetics

BC0663 FUNDAMENTAL PROBLEMS IN BREAST CANCER
International Symposium on Fundamental Problems in Breast
1987, vol. XVIII, p. 407

BC0664 PRIMARY MANAGEMENT OF BREAST CANCER: ALTERNATIVES TO MASTECTOMY
1985, vol. XVII, p. 220
Mastectomy

BC0665 GROWTH FACTORS AND ONCOGENES IN BREAST CANCER
1987
Growth Factors

BC0666 CANCER OF THE BREAST

1988, vol. XII, p. 796

BC0667 BREAST CANCER

1990, vol. 1

BC0668 CELLULAR AND MOLECULAR BIOLOGY OF MAMMARY CANCER

1987, vol. IX, p. 518
Cellular and Molecular Biology

BC0669 BREAST CANCER: COLLABORATIVE MANAGEMENT

1988, vol. XV, p. 390

BC0670 TUMORS OF THE BREAST

53rd Annual Anatomic Pathology Slide Seminar of the American
1988, vol. XI, p. 131

BC0671 BREAST CANCER: CELLULAR AND MOLECULAR BIOLOGY

1988, vol. XVIII, p. 397
Cellular and Molecular Biology

BC0672 BREAST CANCER:SCIENTIFIC AND CLINICAL PROGRESS

International Association for breast Cancer Research
1988, vol. XIX, p. 389

BC0673 PERIODIC SCREENING FOR BREAST CANCER: THE HEALTH INSURANCE PLAN PROJECT AND ITS SEQUELAE, 1963-1986

1988, vol. XIV, p. 214
Health Insurance

BC0674 PROLACTIN AND LESIONS IN BREAST, UTERUS, AND PROSTATE

1989, p. 229
Uterus Cancer, Prolactin; Prostate Cancer

BC0675 WOMEN AT HIGH RISK TO BREAST CANCER

1989, p. 133
Risk Factors

BC0676 BREAST CANCER RATES IN ST. LOUIS PARK: MORTALITY (1960-84) AND INCIDENCE (1981-85) UPDATE

1987, vol. VI, p. 26
St. Louis Park

BC0677 BREAST CANCER

1989, vol. XVI, p. 287

BC0678 BREAST DISEASE FOR GYNECOLOGISTS

1990, vol. XVII, p. 296
Gynecologists

BC0679 INTEGUMENT AND MAMMARY GLANDS

1989, vol. XVI, p. 347

BC0680 BREAST CANCER

1989, vol. X, p. 248

BC0681 THERAPEUTIC MANAGEMENT OF METASTATIC BREAST CANCER

Consensus Development in Cancer Therapy
1989
Metastatic Cancer

BC0682 BREAST CANCER: PROGRESS IN BIOLOGY, CLINICAL MANAGEMENT, AND PREVENTION
Proceedings of the International Association for Breast Cancer
1989, vol. XVI, p. 239

BC0683 CURRENT PERSPECTIVES IN BREAST CANCER
International Symposium on Breast Cancer
1988, vol. XI, p. 298

BC0684 REGULATORY MECHANISMS IN BREAST CANCER: ADVANCES IN CELLULAR AND MOLECULAR BIOLOGY OF BREAST CANCER
Cancer Treatment and Research
1990, vol. XII, p. 452
Regulatory Mechanisms

BC0685 TREATMENT OF EARLY BREAST CANCER
Early Breast Cancer Trialists' Collaborative Group
1990, vol. V
Early cncer

BC0686 THE BREAST: COMPREHENSIVE MANAGEMENT OF BENIGN AND MALIGNANT DISEASES
1991, vol. XXIII, p. 1128

BC0687 BREAST CANCER: TEXTBOOK FOR GENERAL PRACTITIONERS
1990, p. 67

BC0688 HIGH-RISK BREAST CANCER: THERAPY
1991, vol. XII, p. 517

BC0689 BREAST DISEASES
1991, vol. XVI, p. 928

BC0690 WOMEN'S HEALTH
Subcommittee on Health and the Environment
1990, vol. IV, p. 262

BC0691 MECHANISMS OF PROGRESSION TO HORMONE-INDEPENDENT GROWTH OF BREAST AND PROSTATIC CANCER
1991, vol. VIII, p. 200
Prostatic Cancer

BC0692 BREAST CANCER TREATMENT: A COMPREHENSIVE GUIDE TO MANAGEMENT
1991, vol. XXI, p. 647

BC0693 ZNS-METASTASIERUNG DES MAMMAKARZINOMS
1991, vol. X, p. 139

BC0694 WHY ARE WE LOSING THE WAR ON BREAST CANCER?
Committee on Labor and Human Resources
1991, vol. III, p. 70

BC0695 BREAST CANCER: BIOLOGICAL AND CLINICAL PROGRESS
International Association for Breast Cancer Research
1992, vol. XIX, P. 311

BC0696 TEXTBOOK OF BREAST DISEASE
1992, vol. XII, p. 370

BC0697 GENES, ONCOGENES, AND HORMONES: ADVANCES IN CELLULAR AND MOLECULAR BIOLOGY OF BREAST CANCER

1992, vol. XX, p. 446
Hormones

BC0698 GYNECOLOGICAL CANCER

World Congress of Gynecology and Obstetrics

1992
Gynecological Cancer

BC0699 ATLAS OF BREAST CANCER

1993

BC0700 ENZYME, CANCER SPREAD: LINK CONFIRMED

Science News

Feb. 10, 1990, vol. 137, n. n6, p. 92(1)
Enzymes

BC0701 THE INSULIN CONNECTION

Discover

Apr. 1991, vol. 12, n. n4, p. 16(1)
Progesterone

BC0702 OUR BODIES, OUR FIGHT

Glamour

Aug. 1991, vol. 89, n. n8, p. 80(1)
Federal aid to medical research

BC0703 WOMEN WITH BREAST CANCER SPEAK OUT

Vogue

Aug. 1991, vol. 181, n. n8, p. 178(1)

BC0704 A COMPARISON OF TREATMENT OUTCOMES FOR BLACK PATIENTS AND WHITE PATIENTS WITH METASTATIC BREAST CANCER: THE PIEDMONT ONCOLOGY ASSOCIATION EXPERIENCE

The Journal of the American Medical Association

Sept. 18, 1991, vol. 266, n. n11, p. 1494(1)
Black Patients

BC0705 RASHAD JOINS EFFORT TO BATTLE BREAST CANCER

Jet

Nov. 25, 1991, vol. 81, n. n6, p. 5(1)
Health promotion

BC0706 BREAST CANCER: A TABOO TRANSFORMED

U.S. News and World Report

May 11, 1992, vol. 112, n. n18, p. 62(4)
Alternative medicine

BC0707 CHANCE OF BREAST CANCER IS FIGURED AT 1 IN 8

The New York Times

Sept. 27, 1992, vol. 142, p. 13(N) p30
Odds

BC0708 BREAST CANCER

Washington G.A.O.

Dec. 11, 1991, p. 48

BC0709 THE 184 BEST BREAST CANCER DOCTORS

Abrams, M.
Good Housekeeping
Apr. 1989, vol. 208, n. n4, p. 77(6)
Surgeons; Oncologists; Gynecology

BC0710 BREAST CANCER: NEW HOPE IN THE '90'S

Abrams, M.
Good Housekeeping
Oct. 1990, vol. 211, n. n4, p. 77(4)
Oncology; Oncologists

BC0711 REDUCTION TO HOMOZYGOSITY OF GENES ON CHROMOSOME 11 IN HUMAN BREAST NEOPLASIA

Ali, I.U.; R.
Science
Oct. 9, 1987, vol. 238, p. 185(4)
Carcinogenesis; oncogenes; DNA

RFLP analysis of loci on chromosome 11 in breast cancer patients. Constitutional and tumor genotypes of markers on chromosome 11. Analysis of polymorphic markers on chromosome 11 and other autosomes. Schematic representation of the deletions on short arm of chromosome 11. Loss of constitutional heterozygosity of loci on chromosome 11. Correlation between chromosome 11p depletion and histopathological parameters.

BC0712 OUR BODIES, THEIR SELVES: A BIAS AGAINST WOMEN IN HEALTH RESEARCH

Ames, K. and L.
Newsweek
Dec. 17, 1990, vol. 116, n. n25, p. 60(1)
Cardiovascular diseases; Osteoporosis; Chlamydia; AIDS (disease)

BC0713 BREAST CANCER

Barner, W.
Science and Technology Division
1991, p. 16

BC0714 THE POLITICS OF BREAST CANCER: FIRST THEY CRIED. THEN THEY GO MAD. NOW VICTIMS ARE TAKING THEIR BATTLES INTO THE COURTS AND INTO THE STREETS

Beck, M. and L.
Newsweek
Dec. 10, 1990, vol. 116, n. n24, p. 62(3)
Mammography; Bone marrow
Dollars for diseases. (table)

BC0715 IN RESEARCH WOMEN DON'T MATTER
Berney, B.
Progressive
Oct. 1990, vol. 54, p. 24-27
Women; Research

BC0716 LOSS OF HETEROZYGOSITY ON CHROMOSOME 7Q AND AGGRESSIVE PRIMARY BREAST CANCER
Bieche, I.
The Journal of the American Medical Association
Apr. 1, 1992, vol. 267, n. n13, p. 1745(1)
Chromosome 7Q

BC0717 A SWITCH IN TIME SAVES A STATISTICAL BIND
Blume, E.; C.T.
The Journal of the American Medical Association
Dec. 18, 1991, vol. 266, n. n23, p. 3284(2)

BC0718 MOM'S DON'T GET SICK
Brack, P. and B.
Ladies' Home Journal
Aug. 1190, vol. 107, n. n8, p. 76(4)

BC0719 LIFE WISH: ONE WOMAN'S STRUGGLE AGAINST MEDICAL INCOMPETENCE
Carroll, P.
1986, vol. XII, p. 204
Thyroid gland; Surgical errors

BC0720 BREAST CARCINOMA METASTATIC TO THE UVEA
Catalano, R.A.; D.
The Journal of the American Medical Association
Aug. 22, 1990, vol. 264, n. n8, p. 1032(1)
Uvea
A 45-year-old female patient complained of decreasing vision; she had a malignant tumor (adenocarcinoma) of the breast one year before. During an eye examination, a yellow mass accompanied by pigment was detected beneath, and partially detaching, the retina of both eyes. A 57-year-old woman who also had breast cancer was examined for visual problems as well. In this case, a white fluffy mass was visible in the anterior chamber of the eye, partially obscuring the iris and pupil. A diagnosis of metastatic spread to the middle, vascular layer of the eye (the uvea) was made in both cases. Although considered rare, approximately 38 percent of all symptoms of visual impairment, and 9 percent of women without visual symptoms had metastasis to the uvea after breast cancer. Breast cancer is three times more likely to spread to the eye than other forms of cancer; the reason for this is unknown. Radiation, often without the use of chemotherapy, can be used to control this metastasis, but the average survival time after uvula metastases is only nine months. (Consumer Summary produced by Reliance Medical Information, Inc.) Fundus photograph of left eye showing yellow mass. (diagnostic image) Direct slit-lamp exam shows fluff-appearing white mass. (diagnostic image)

BC0721 QUALITY OF CARE-TIME TO ACT

Chassin, M.R.
The Journal of the American Medical Association
Dec. 25, 1991, vol. 266, n. n24, p. 3472(2)
Medical research

The development of new quality assessment tools has led to more objective measurements of the quality of care in the medical field. Increasingly, problems are being identified in the quality of care provided in the U. S. These problems can be placed into three general categories: overuse, underuse, and misuse of medical care. Overuse is when risks of a health service outweigh benefits; underuse if when benefits outweigh risks, yet the service is not used; and misuse is when the service itself is improperly performed. In the December 25, 1991 issue of The Journal of the American Medical Association, two articles are presented that show how registry data can be used to study underuse. The first study by hand and colleagues used breast cancer data from a cancer registry to examine if treatments proven effective in treating breast cancer were being properly utilized by hospitals. Their results showed that some of the treatments were not being fully utilized and observed certain characteristics of hospitals that were failing to properly utilize these treatments. In the second article by Lazovich and colleagues, breast cancer treatment data were again examined. The study examined if conservative surgery, which is now recommended for early-stage breast cancer, was generally being used, and if radiation therapy (which should accompany conservative surgery) was also being used. The results revealed that many women with early-stage breast cancer did not receive conservative surgery, despite the fact that only a small portion of the women were ineligible for conservative surgery. Radiation therapy was to given to 14 percent of the women who receive conservative surgery. Both studies raised quality of care issues. Further research is needed to discover how and where quality of care was compromised for these patients. The research methodologies for these types of studies also need further refinement, but both reports show that objective assessments of quality of care are now available. (Consumer Summary produced by Reliance Medical Information. Inc.)

BC0722 BREAST CANCER: MINIMALISTS, MAXIXALISTS, OTHER NEOPLASMS

Cohen, M.H.; R.G.
The Journal of the American Medical Association
May 22, 1991, vol. 265, n. n20, p. 2668(3)
Medical Screening

Surveillance arms in two randomized clinical trials. (table)

BC0723 COUNTDOWN TO THE CURE: HOW TEXANS ARE FIGHTING THE WAR AGAINST BREAST CANCER: SUSAN G. KOMEN FOUNDATION

Connatser, J.; S.
Texas Monthly
Oct. 1990, vol. 18, n. n10, p. 69(17)
Medical research

Facts about breast cancer. (table)

BC0724 A BOON OR BUST FOR WOMEN? FDA'S HEARING ON BREAST IMPLANTS ENDS IN DRAW

Cowley, G.
Newsweek
Nov. 25, 1991, vol. 118, n. n22, p. 65(1)
Silicones in medicine; Breast diseases

BC0725 BREAST CANCER RISK FACTORS AND SCREENING: UNITED STATES, 1987

Dawson, D.A.

1990, vol. IV, p. 60
Risk Factors; Screening

BC0726 "I CAN'T HAVE BREAST CANCER - I'M ONLY 35!"

Dawson, M.
Ladies' Home Journal

Nov. 1989, vol. 106, n. n11, p. 104(6)

BC0727 ESTROGEN-INDUCED FACTORS OF BREAST CANCER CELLS PARTIALLY REPLACE ESTROGEN TO PROMOTE TUMOR GROWTH

Dickson, R.B;
Science

June 20, 1986, vol. 232, p. 1540(4)
Estrogen
Growth factors and estradiol in development of human breast cancers in mice. Dose dependence of CME2 activity. Time dependence of CME2 activity

BC0728 8 DANGEROUS BREAST CANCER MYTHS

Dowden, R. and J.
Redbook

May 1990, vol. 175, n. n1, p. 114(2)
Medical misconceptions

BC0729 HELPING HANDS

Doyle-Driedger, S.
Maclean's

Mar. 30, 1992, vol. 105, n. n13, p. 42(1)

BC0730 UNRAVELING CANCER'S SECRETS

Dranov, P.
Ladies' Home Journal

Oct. 1992, vol. 109, n. n10, p. 97(8)
Ovarian cancer; Colorectal cancer

BC0731 THE INDIVIDUAL VS SOCIETY: IS THERE A CONFLICT

Eddy, D.M.
The Journal of the American Medical Association

Mar. 20, 1991, vol. 265, n. n11, p. 1446(3)
Medical care, cost of
Health and economic outcomes of two health plans. (table)

BC0732 BEATING BREAST CANCER: RESEARCHERS ARE LOOKING BEYOND CONVENTIONAL SURGERIES AND CHEMOTHERAPY

Edwards, D.D.
Science News

May 14, 1988, vol. 133, n. n20, p. 314(2)
Tamoxifen; estrogen; preoperative care; mastectomy

BC0733 GONADOTROPIN-RELEASING HORMONE BINDING SITES IN HUMAN BREAST CARCINOMA

Eidne, KA..; C.A.
Science

Sept. 6, 1985, vol. 229, p. 989(3)
Hormone receptors; Immunochemistry
Ligand immunoblot analysis of solubilized breast tumor membranes. Displacement of GnRH bound to human ductal breast tumor membranes.. GnRH receptors in relation to histological classification and estrogen and progesterone receptors in women.

BC0734 BREAST CANCER RISK LINKED TO DENSE TISSUE

Fackelmann, K.A.
Science News
Apr. 8, 1989, vol. 135, n. n14, p. 213(1)
Risk; Tissue

BC0735 FRONT-PAGE CANCER NEWS TELL ONLY PART OF THE STORY

Feldman, M.
Mpls. St. Paul
Apr. 1992, vol. 20, n. n4, p. 25(1)

BC0736 WHAT'S NEXT IN TREATMENT

Fraser, L.
Vogue
Oct. 1992, vol. 182, n. n10, p. 331(2)
Treatments

BC0737 A QUESTION OF LIFE

Frenkiel, N.
The New York Times Magazine
May 3, 1992, vol. 141, p. 36

BC0738 TREATMENT OPTIONS FOR BREAST CANCER-BEYOND SURVIVAL

Ganz, P.A.
The New England Journal of Medicine
Apr. 23, 1992, vol. 326, n. n17, p. 1147(3)
Mastectomy; Lumpectomy; Informed consent (Medical law)

Advances in the understanding of breast cancer have changed treatment options for women with early stage breast cancer. Many of these women can be treated with breast-conserving surgery such as a lumpectomy, quadrantectomy or partial mastectomy rather than a radical mastectomy. Two research studies found that breast-conserving surgery is used to treat woman with early-stage breast cancer most often in the Northeast U. S., least often in the Southeast U. S. and most often in the 17 states with informed consent laws. The use of breast-conserving surgery also was related to the type of hospital at which the patient was treated. These studies also found that use of breast-conserving surgery was lower in older women, and fewer older women who had breast-conserving surgery had radiation therapy. Surgeons' beliefs and practice methods, especially in providing information on treatment options, may affect the use of breast-conserving therapy. The effect of a radical mastectomy on a woman's quality of life should be weighed against the threat of cancer recurrence.

BC0739 FIGHTING FOR THEIR LIVES: THE LARGER GOOD

Goode, E.E.
U.S. News and World Report
Aug. 26, 1991, vol. 111, n. n9, p. 68(2)
Elenore Pred. (portrait)

BC0740 PATTERNS OF CARE RELATED TO AGE OF BREAST CANCER PATIENTS

Greenfield, S.; Blanco; Elashoff; Ganz, P.A.
JAMA: The Journal of the American Medical Association
May 22, 1987, vol. 257, p. 2766(5)
Geriatric oncology

Comorbidity index and criteria map: reliability studies. Hospital characteristics. The relation of age to stage at initial presentation. Breast cancer treat ment score. The relation of the comorbidity index to physical management of breast cancer. Effect of age, comorbidity, and hospital on appropriate treatment. Relationship of age to proportion of patients with appropriate treatment. Appropriate treatment for patients in stage I and II.

BC0741 TURN APPLES INTO PEARS

Gutfield, G.
Prevention
Dec, 1991, vol. 43, n. n12, p. 9(2)
Reducing diets

BC0742 LINKAGE OF EARLY-ONSET FAMILIAL BREAST CANCER TO CHROMOSOME 17Q21

Hall, J.M.; M.K.
Science
Dec. 21, 1990, vol. 250, n. n4988, p. 1684(6)
Tumor suppressor genes

Certain diseases, including some forms of breast cancer, are inherited. The inherited form of breast cancer occurs at an earlier age, frequently involves both breasts, and occurs in men more often than the non-inherited form of breast cancer. Studies of certain genetic sequences, known as genetic markers, which are inherited along with the disease, have allowed the identification of the site on the chromosomes (structural units where the genes are located) where the genetic defect lies. These studies can lead to the identification of the gene that is directly involved in the disease process. A gene involved the susceptibility of the inherited form of breast cancer was localized to the q21 position of chromosome 17.

BC0743 ASSESSING THE RISK OF RECURRENCE IN BREAST CANCER

Ingle, J.N.
The New England Journal of Medicine
Feb. 1, 1990, vol. 322, n. n5, p. 329(3)
Cathepsin D; Estrogen; Lymph Nodes

The search for even better methods of predicting the prognosis of a cancer patient is at the forefront of today's cancer research. An article in the February 1, 1990 issue of 'The New England Journal of Medicine' presents the results of assessing the risk for the recurrence of breast cancer by a relatively simple test. The ability to predict which patients with breast disease are likely to be at high risk for cancer recurrence would be important in planning clinical treatment. In 1979, a glycoprotein (combination of protein and carbohydrate) was identified as being secreted by human breast cancer cells grown in laboratory tissue cultures. After purification this molecule, called cathepsin D, was identified as a precursor of an enzyme which acts to break down protein (i.e., a protease). This compound was found to be stimulated by the level of female hormones or estrogens, and its level was restricted by anti-estrogen drugs (which oppose estrogens).

BC0744 WHAT YOU SHOULD KNOW ABOUT MALE CANCERS

Jabs, C.
Woman's Day
Aug. 19, 1986, p. 27(3)
Prostate cancer

BC0745 REQUIREMENT FOR THE ADENOVIRUS TYPE 9 E4 REGION IN PRODUCTION OF MAMMARY TUMORS

Javier, R.; K.
Science
Aug. 28, 1992, vol. 257, n. n5074, p. 1267(5)
Oncogenic viruses

BC0746 TRANSFECTION OF V-RASH DNA INTO MCF-7 HUMAN BREAST CANCER CELLS BYPASSES DEPENDENCE ON ESTROGEN FOR TUMORIGENICITY

Kasid, A. Lippman, Parageorge, Lowry, D.R. et al.
Science
May 10, 1985, vol. 228, p. 725(4)
Estrogen; DNA

Total cellular E2 and progesterone specific receptor concentrations. Effects of estrogen and antiestrogen on thymidine incorporation in growth-arrested cells. Effects of E2 and antiestrogen on cell proliferation of wild-type and transfected MCF-7 cells. Tumor growth in the nude mice.

BC0747 EPIDEMIOLOGY OF BREAST CANCER

Kelsey, J.L. and
Epidemiologic Reviews
1990, vol. 12, p. 228-240
Epidemiology

BC0748 PROLACTIN AND BREAST CANCER

Kleinberg, D.L.
The New England Journal of Medicine
Jan. 29, 1987, vol. 316, p. 269(3)
Prolactin

BC0749 ONCOGENES GIVE BREAST CANCER PROGNOSIS; AMPLIFICATION OF AN ONCOGENE IN BREAST CANCER CELLS CORRELATES WITH TIME TO RELAPSE AND SURVIVAL TIME.

Kolata, G.
Science
Jan. 9, 1987, vol. 235, p. 160(2)
Oncogenic viruses

BC0750 RACE FOR THE CURE

Kowalchik, C.
Runner's World
July 1991, vol. 26, n. n7, p. 52(9)
Cures
Nancy Brinker. (portrait)

BC0751 HAPTOGLOBIN-RELATED PROTEIN (HRP) EPITOPES IN BREAST CANCER AS A PREDICTOR OF RECURRENCE OF THE DISEASE

Kuhajda, F.P.; S.
The New England Journal of Medicine
Sept. 7, 1989, vol. 321, n. n10, p. 636(5)
Haptoglobin-Related Protein Epitopes
The ability to assess the likelihood of the spread of cancer, metastatic activity, at the time of the initial diagnosis of breast cancer would be an important component in selecting patients for intensive early chemotherapy. Currently, more than 25 percent of patients have undetectable metastases in the early stages of breast cancer. Studies show a relationship between changes in oncogenes, gene viruses that can cause cells to become malignant, and possible outcomes of breast cancer. Some human breast cancer oncogenes that shares epitopes (a component of an antigen, a molecule capable of producing disease) with the HPR gene product. Researchers studied the activity of HPR-epitopes in early cancer tissues from human breasts and concluded that the expression of HPR-epitopes can be used to predict metastasis in patients with early breast cancer. Approximately 45 percent to 92 percent of patients exhibiting Hpr has recurrence of cancer, while 22 percent of those not exhibiting Hpr had recurrence. Analysis of Hpr would be useful in assessing the treatment options available to patients with early breast cancer. It may also be useful o measure blood levels of Hpr in monitoring the progression of the disease in high risk patients.

BC0752 8 MEDICAL MIRACLES FROM NATURE: THEY'RE UNUSUAL, THEY'RE ALMOST UNHEARD OF, BUT THE EVIDENCE SO FAR IS IN THEIR FAVOR

Lally, S.
Prevention
Nov. 1989, vol. 41, n. n11, p. 33(9)
; Transcutaneous electrical nerve stimulation; tobacco; AIDS; Melanoma; Vaccine; Ovarian cancers; Taxol; Implants, artificial;

BC0753 IS THERE A DOCTOR (OF WOMEN'S HEALTH) IN THE HOUSE?

Lamb, L.
UTNE Reader
Mar.-Apr. 1992, n. n50, p. 26(2)

BC0754 BREAST CANCER

Laurence, L.
Working Woman
Sept. 1992, vol. 17, n. n9, p. 91(3)

BC0755 INACTIVATION OF THE RETINOBLASTOMA SUSCEPTIBILITY GENE IN HUMAN BREAST CANCERS
Lee, E.Y.; H. To; J.
Science
July 8, 1988, vol. 241, n. n4862, p. 218(4)
Mutagenesis
Structure of mutant RB genes from the normal RB gene map.

BC0756 A PROSPECTIVE STUDY OF BENIGN BREAST DISEASE AND THE RISK OF BREAST CANCER
London, S.J.; J.
Journal of the American Medical Association
Feb. 19, 1992, vol. 267, p. 941-944

BC0757 UNDERGROUND MEDICINE
Lord, M.
U.S. News and World Report
May 11, 1992, vol. 112, n. n18, p. 62(4)
Alternative medicine; Alzheimer's disease; AIDS (disease); Lyme disease

BC0758 BREAST CANCER: STALEMATE IN THE WAR ON CANCER
Marshall, E.
Science
Dec. 20 ,1991, vol. 254, n. n 5039, p. 1719(2)

BC0759 CELL GROWTH CONTROL TAKES BALANCE: THE UNCONTROLLED DIVISION OF CANCER MAY RESULT EITHER FROM EXCESSIVE GROWTH STIMULATION OR DEFICIENT GROWTH INHIBITION
Marx, J.L.
Science
Feb. 26, 1988, vol. 239, n. n4843, p. 975(2)
Cell proliferation

BC0760 GENE SIGNALS RELAPSE OF BREAST, OVARIAN CANCERS
Marx, J.L.
Science
May 12, 1989, vol. 244, n. n4905, p. 654(2)
Amplification

BC0761 STRETCH EXERCISE PROGRAM: A PROGRAM FOR WOMEN WHO HAVE HAD BREAST CANCER
McGee-Colburn, J.
1988, vol. XVIII, p.
Stretch Exercise Program

BC0762 JEDEN TAG WILL ICH LEBEN: EIN KREBSTAGEBUCH
Mechtel, A.
1990, p. 159

BC0763 CLINICAL ALERT GIVES BREAST CANCER DATA, REVISES RECOMMENDATIONS
Merz, B.
JAMA: The Journal of the American Medical Associations
July 8, 1988, vol. 260, n. n2, p. 153(2)

BC0764 SHORT-CIRCUITING ONCOGENES MAY BECOME BASIS OF NEW CANCER THERAPIES

Merz, B.
The Journal of the American Medical Association
Nov. 24, 1989, vol. 262, n. n20, p. 2785(1)
Carcinogenesis
Oncogenes are a normal genetic component of all human cells. These genes may have a role in the process of cellular proliferation that occurs in normal growth and that leads to tumor formation. Speakers at the 12th Annual Bristol-Myers Symposium on Cancer Research (held in Toronto, Canada) discussed how proteins produced as the result of the expression of oncogenes may have a variety of physiologic functions which, with understanding, may be used to stop, regress or even prevent the development of cancers. This concept appears valid when one considers that the oncogenes carry the genetic information for producing approximately 60 different proteins, each with a normal cell function. In part, this concept is derived from the work of a group of investigators, including J. Michael Bishop and Howard Varmus, who will shortly receive a Nobel Prize for his work. Oncogenes appear to be involved in several general classifications: phosphorylation, growth and deoxyribonucleic acid (DNA) replication. Their work has also shown that each of these groups of oncogenes produce products that function best in specific areas of the cell. (For example, the myc protein controls messenger-RNA and is found in the cell nucleus.) When the genes become altered, their protein products are similarly disturbed. A protein product normally attached to the cell membrane could be increased in concentration and found in an unusual area of a cell. Although this process by itself is unlikely to lead to malignancy, when coupled with other similar changes, a cancer could develop. A possible direction of therapy could be to prevent such events. Other areas of research concentrate on the environment in which cancer formation occurs. The rate of breast cancer is higher in women who have induce the changes in the breast that occur as a result of pregnancy in childless women. This research points to changing the biochemical environment instead of removing or altering genes.

BC0765 BREAST CANCER

Morra, M. and E.
Good Housekeeping
May 1987, vol. 204, p. 153(4)

BC0766 CANCER: THE ISSUE FEMINISTS FORGOT

Neuman, E.
Insight (Washington Times)
Feb. 9, 1992, vol. 8, p. 7-11, 24-26
Federal aid to medical research

BC0767 CANCER: THE ISSUE FEMINISTS FORGOT

Neuman, E.
Insight
Feb. 24, 1992, vol. 8, n. n8, p. 6(9)

BC0768 GENES OF WAR

Noonan, D.
Discover
Oct. 1990,vol. 11, p. 46-52
Genetic research; research; DNA

BC0769 GENES OF WAR; ARMED ONLY WITH TINY FRAGMENTS OF DNA

Noonan, D.
Discover
Oct. 1990, vol. 11, n. n10, p. 46(7)
HLA histocompatibility antigens; Mitochondrial DNA; DNA fingerprints
Mary-Claire King. (portrait) Mitochondrial DNA appears as a convoluted loop. (chart) Mitochondrial DNA helps reunite children of Argentina's disappeared. (chart)

BC0770 FIGHTING THE BREAST CANCER PANIC

Payer, L.
Vogue
Oct. 1992, vol. 182, n. n10, p. 328(5)
Mammography

BC0771 BREAST CANCER IN A MALE-TO-FEMALE TRANSSEXUAL; A CASE REPORT

Pritchard, T.J.;
JAMA: The Journal of the American Medical Associations
Apr. 15, 1988, vol. 259, n. n15, p. 2278(3)
Transsexuals

BC0772 NO MORE WAITING

Quindlen, A.
The New York Times Magazine
July 22, 1992, vol. 141, p. A13(N) pA1
Mifepristone; Medical policy

BC0773 HYPERTENSION IN PREGNANCY CUTS CANCER RISK

Raloff, J.
Science News
Oct. 21, 1989, vol. 136, n. n17, p. 263(1)
Alpha Fetoproteins

BC0774 ENZYME SUGGESTS BREAST CANCER SPREAD

Raloff, J.
Science News
Nov. 18, 1989, vol. 136, n. n21, p. 325(1)
Enzyme Testing

BC0775 TREATMENT OF ADVANCED CARCINOMA OF THE BREAST IN THE MALE

Renziehausen, L.
The Journal of the American Medical Association
June 3, 1992, vol. 267, n. n21, p. 2878(1)
Chemotherapy; Hormone therapy

BC0776 BREAST CANCER-ASSOCIATED PS2 PROTEIN: SYNTHESIS AND SECRETION BY NORMAL STOMACH MUCOSA

Rio, M.C.; J.P.
Science
Aug. 5, 1988, vol. 241, n n4866, p. 705(4)
Protein research
Presence of pS2 immunoreactive material in gastric fluid. Characterization of pS2 mRNA in normal stomach antrum. Comparison of the amino acid sequence of pS2 protein from amino acids 31-84.

BC0777 BREAST CANCER POLITICS
Rochman, S.
The Progressive
Nov. 1991, vol. 55, n. n11, p. 12(1)
Politcal Aspects

BC0778 BREAST CANCER CARE: KNOWING YOUR OPTIONS
Rosenfeld, I.
Vogue
Oct. 1992, vol. 182, n. n10, p. 230(1)

BC0779 NEW CHOICES: THE LATEST OPTIONS IN TREATING BREAST CANCER
Rubenstein, M.
1985, p. 211
Treatmen

BC0780 HEREDITARY BREAST-CANCER PRECAUTIONS
Sandmaier, M.
Mademoiselle
Nov. 1989, vol. 95, n. n11, p. 144(1)
Hereditary Cancer

BC0781 APPLICATIONS OF DIFFUSION THEORY TO CANCER CARE IN THE UNITED STATES, 1972-1981
Schoenfeld, E.R.
1989, vol. VII, p. 156
Diffusion Theory

BC0782 A 43-YEAR OLD WOMAN WITH BREAST CANCER AND THE ABRUPT ONSET OF RESPIRATORY FAILURE
Scully, R.E.; E.J.
The New England Journal of Medicine
July 23, 1987
Metastasis

BC0783 A 57-YEAR-OLD WOMAN WITH WORSENING OPSOCLONUS
Scully, R.E.; E.J.
The New England Journal of Medicine
Mar. 1988, vol. 13, n. n5, p. 1(4)

BC0784 AN 82-YEAR OLD WOMAN WITH A COMPLETE LEFT FACIAL PALSY AND A LEFT MASTOID MASS
Scully, R.E.; E.J.
The New England Journal of Medicine
Apr. 6, 1989, vol. 320, n. n14, p. 924(7)
Adenocarcinoma; Temporal Bone

BC0785 INDICATORS OF PROGNOSIS IN NODE-NEGATIVE BREAST CANCER

Sigurdsson, H.; B.
The New England Journal of Medicine
Apr. 12, 1990, vol. 322, n. n15, p. 1045(9)
Node-Negative Cancer
Studies of survival after the diagnosis of breast cancer suggest that patients fall into two groups, in terms of potential for cancer recurrence. Women in one group suffer from breast cancer that is rapidly fatal, while women in the other group have a survival rate that is similar to that of women without beast cancer. The majority of patients who breast cancer is node-negative, meaning it has not spread to the lymph nodes, can simply have the tumor removed and will never experience recurrence. More breast cancer patients are expected to have this positive outcome, as improved screening methods are being used to diagnose the disease earlier. It has been predicted that over 50 percent of patients with a new diagnosis of breast cancer will be found to have node-negative cancer. Prognostic indicators are needed for categorizing women with node-negative cancer into those who should have systemic therapy, such as chemotherapy, after surgery and those who do not need it. Women at greater risk for recurrence should be identified and given the adjuvant (additional) therapy, while those at lower risk may not benefit from such treatment and may be harmed by the side effects. A group of 367 Swedish women with node-negative breast cancer were studied to identify prognostic indicators. All had the tumors surgical removed, and 83 women (28 percent) also receive adjuvant therapy, which was tamoxifen in most cases, Different characteristics of the patients and their tumors were evaluated for their association with prognosis. Three useful indicators were identified; these were tumor size, progesterone-receptor status, and S-phase fraction, a characteristic of the tumor cells. Using these three indicators in a prognostic model, the subjects were divided into two groups: 37 percent of subjects were classified as high-risk for a delayed recurrence of cancer and the other 63 percent were low-risk. The low-risk group had a five-year overall survival rate of 92 percent, which did not differ from that of other Swedish women of the same ages. A prognostic index such as the one used here, which indicated the proliferative activity of the tumor cells, may be able to identify those patients with node-negative breast cancer who are at low-risk for recurrence and can safely avoid chemotherapy. (Consumer Summary produced by Reliance Medical Information, Inc.) Characteristics and treatment of patients with breast cancer. (table) Univariate analysis of prognostic covariates. (table) Overall survival and survival with breast cancer. (graph) Multivariate analysis of prognostic covariates of survival. (table) Cumulative survival according to pattern of risk factors. (table) Survival according to defined risk group. (graph) Overall survival according to number of risk factors. (graph)

BC0786 GENETIC CLUE TO CANCER PROGNOSIS

Silberner, J.
Science News
Jan. 17, 1987, vol. 131, p. 46(1)
Genetics

BC0787 CONQUERING PROSTATE CANCER

Silberner, J.
U.S. News and World Report
July 10, 1989, vol. 107, n. n2, p. 55(3)
Prostate Cancer
Two prostate solutions. (chart) Prostate vs. breast cancer. (table) The man-killing cancer. (table)

BC0788 AFFORDING BREAST-CANCER TREATMENT

Silver, M.; C.
U.S. News and World Report
dec. 3, 1990, vol. 109, n. n22, p.79(1)
Autografts; Insurance

BC0789 INHERITANCE OF PROLIFERATIVE BREAST DISEASE IN BREAST CANCER KINDRED

Skolnick, M.H.;
Science
Dec. 21, 1990, vol. 250, n. n4988, p. 1715(6)

Certain types of breast cancer are inherited, and some individual s have up to 10 times the risk of developing breast cancer because of a genetic predisposition. This study shows that patients with proliferative breast disease (PBD) may also have an increased risk of developing breast cancer. PBD is characterized by noncancerous growth of epithelial cells of the ducts of the breasts. The association between PBD and breast cancer was studied in 103 women (among 20 different families with two first-degree relatives with breast cancer, and in 31 control women without a family history of breast cancer. Physical examinations, mammography, and needle aspirates from breast tissue were performed on all subjects. Analysis of breast tissue showed that 35 percent of the women with a family history of breast cancer, but who were clinically normal, had PBD, while only 13 percent of the women without a family history of breast cancer had PBD. The study concluded that individuals could be genetically susceptible to PBD and breast cancer, and provides evidence for the current theory that several genetic changes are necessary for the progression to cancer. (Consumer Summary produced by Reliance Medical Information. Inc.) Twenty pedigrees used to study the occurrence of breast cancer. (chart) Samples for cytological examination. (diagnostic image) Parameter estimates for genetic models. (table) Frequency of detection of PBD in first degree relatives. (table) Linkage analysis with D17S74. (table)

BC0790 HUMAN BREAST CANCER: CORRELATION OF RELAPSE AND SURVIVAL WITH AMPLIFICATION OF THE HER-2-NEU ONCOGENE

Slamon, D.J. ; G.
Science
Jan. 9, 1987, vol. 235, p. 177(6)
Cell division

Assn. between HER-2-neu amplification and disease parameter Univariate, multivariate analyses of survival, relapse, in node-pos. patient Actuarial curve for relapse in node positive patients.

BC0791 STUDIES OF THE HER-2-NEU PROTO-ONCOGENE IN HUMAN BREAST AND OVARIAN CANCER

Slamon, D.J.; W.
Science
May 12, 1989, vol. 244, n. n4905, p. 707(6)
Gene amplification; Gene expression; Carcinogenesis

Multivariate survival analyses comparing survival to prognostic factors. (table) Median survival time and various degrees of HER-2-neu gene expression. (table) Actuarial survival curves, association of gene amplification and survival. (graph)

BC0792 TOP MEDICAL NEWS OF 1989
Slom, C.
McCall's
Dec. 1989, vol. 117, n. n3, p. 97(1)
AIDS (disease); Oral contraceptives; Mammography; Menopause; Human genome initiative

BC0793 BUILDING A WEAPON AGAINST BREAST CANCER
Smith, E.T.
Business Week
Apr. 7, 1986, vol. 293, p. 93(1)
Genetic engineering

BC0794 BREAST CANCER; NEW FORMS OF SUPPORT
Spear, R.
New York
May, 30, 1988, vol. 21, n. n22, p. 26(1)

BC0795 BREAST CANCER: HOW TO DEFEND YOURSELF
Squires, S.
Ladies' Home Journal
Nov. 1988, vol. 105, n. n11, p. 180(7)

BC0796 INDEPENDENT MOLECULAR PATHWAYS IN INITIATION AND LOSS OF HORMONE RESPONSIVENESS OF BREAST CARCINOMAS
Sukumar, S.; W.P.
Science
Apr. 22, 1988, vol. 240, n. n4851, p. 524(3)
Oncogenes; cellular control mechanisms
Expressions of p21 valine in transfected MCF-7 cells. H-ras oncogenes in rat mammary tumors of known hormonal status. Growth properties of MCF-7 cells transfected with H-ras oncogenes.

BC0797 INCIDENCE OF CANCER IN 161 FAMILIES AFFECTED BY ATAXIATELANGIECTASIA
Swift, M.; D. D. Morrell;
The New England Journal of Medicine
Dec. 26, 1991, vol. 325, n. n26, p. 1831(6)
Genetic disorders
Ataxia-telangiectasia is a genetic disorder, inherited as a recessive trait. Patients who are homozygous, that is, who carry two copies of the gene, develop ataxia starting in childhood. This defect in coordinated movement progresses to complete disability by 10 years. Patients with this disorder also develop telangiectasia, or swelling of tiny blood vessels. These telangiectatic lesions generally develop at about three or four years of age. Retrospective studies have indicated that homozygotes are about 100 times more likely to develop cancer than the general population. A prospective study was therefore conducted on 161 families with ataxia-telangiectasia.

BC0798 STRUCTURAL REARRANGEMENT OF THE RETINOBLASTOMA GENE IN HUMAN BREAST CARCINOMA
T'Ang, A.; J.M.
Science
Oct. 14, 1988, vol. 242, n. n4876, p. 263(4)
Mutation (biology); chromosome abnormalities; genetic polymorphisms
Structural aberrations of the RB1 gene in human breast tumors and cell lines. DNA blot analysis of primary human breast tumor samples and cell lines. RNA blot analysis of tumor cell lines.

BC0799 CATHEPSIN D AND PROGNOSIS IN BREAST CANCER

Tandon, A.K.;
The New England Journal of Medicine
Feb. 1, 1990, vol. 322, n. n5, p. 297(6)
Cathepsin D
The ability to predict which patients with breast cancer are likely to be a high risk for recurrence of the disease could be important in planning the clinical treatment of these patients. In 1979 a glycoprotein (combination of protein and carbohydrate) was identified as being secreted by human breast cancer cells grown in laboratory tissue cultures. After purification the molecule, called cathepsin D, was identified as the precursor of an enzyme which acts to break down a protein (i.e., a protease). It was found that this compound is stimulated by the level of female hormones or estrogens, and its level was restricted by anti-estrogen drugs (which opposed estrogens). A classification system for the prognosis of breast cancer patients is related to the degree of cancerous involvement of the lymph nodes; no involvement indicates a better prognosis, and cancer spread to lymph nodes carries a poorer prognosis. In this experiment, tissues taken from 199 mode-positive and 198 node-negative breast cancer patients were analyzed for the level of cathepsin D. The level of this compound was found to be a good predictor of the rate of recurrence in women who were ode-negative, but not in those patients who were node-positive. In node-negative women the level of cathepsin D corresponded to the irregular number of chromosomes present within tumor cells (aneuploidy). Women with a high level of cathepsin D had a rate of recurrence which was 2.6 times greater than those having a low level. Cathepsin D may be useful in identifying women who have an elevated risk of cancer recurrence, and therefore require more aggressive therapy. (Consumer Summary produced by Reliance Medical Information, Inc.) Western blot analysis of cathepsin D in tumor specimens. (chart) Concentration of cathepsin D in breast tumors. (graph) Disease-free survival in patients with breast cancer. (graph) Overall survival in patients with breast cancer. (graph).

BC0800 PATHOLOGY OF THE BREAST

Tavassoli, F.A.
1992, vol. XIII, p. 669
Pathology

BC0801 MEDICINE'S PACK RATS PRODUCE RESULTS: COLLECTIONS

Thomas, P.
Medical World News
July 11, 1986, vol. 29, p. 32-34, 39-42
Acquired immune deficiency syndrome; hereditary diseases; blood

BC0802 MY BREAST: ONE WOMEN'S CANCER STORY

Wadler, J.
New York
Apr. 13, 1992, vol. 37, P. 37-47

BC0803 A PUZZLING PLAGUE

Wallis, C.
Time
Jan 14,1991, vol. 137, p. 48-55
Epidemiology

BC0804 A PUZZLING PLAGUE: WHAsT IS IT ABOUT THE AMERICAN WAY OF LIFE THAT CAUSES BREAST CANCER?

Wallis, C.
Time
Jan. 14, 1991, vol. 137, n. n2, p. 48(5)
America
Incidence of breast cancer per 100,000 U.S. women. (graph) How the risk shapes up. (graph) Where cancer is most likely to be found. (chart) Danger in the diet. (graph)

BC0805 MALPRACTICE DEFENSE: BREAST CANCER

Watts, C.F.
1990, vol. X, p. 195
Malpractice

BC0806 NEW BREAST-CANCER GUIDELINES

Weber, M.
Vogue
Sept. 1988, vol. 178, n. n9, p. 475(1)
New Breasts

BC0807 TUMOR ANGIOGENESIS AND METASTASIS-CORRELATION IN INVASIVE BREAST CANCER

Weidner, N.; J.P.
The New England Journal of Medicine
Jan. 3, 1991, vol. 324, n. n1, p. 1(8)
tumor Angiogenesis; Metastasis
The growth and development of a cancer involves a broad spectrum of events. One key event is the stimulation of new blood vessels which penetrate the tumor and supply it with increased amounts of oxygen and nutrients. Current estimates suggest that early cancers grow slowly and are relatively dormant. When they reach about a million cells (which represents a tumor of only a few millimeters) further growth can not occur without the development of new blood vessels to vascularize the tumor. In addition to providing improved blood supply to the tiny tumor, the new blood vessels provide routes for metastatic cells to crawl out of the primary tumor and circulate to distant parts of the body. A study of 49 breast cancers was undertaken to determine if the number of blood vessels within the tumor correlates with metastatic disease in the patients. Of the 49 patients, 30 had metastatic disease and 19 did not. If the notion that more blood vessels provide more opportunity for metastatic is correct, then more blood vessels would be with metastatic disease. This is precisely what was observed. Researchers without knowledge of the patient's history counted blood vessels under the microscope in tissue sections of breast cancer specimens. An average of 101 blood vessels could be seen in a high power field of the microscope among the patients with metastatic disease. Among patients without metastatic disease, an average of 45 blood vessels were observed. These results confirm the importance of vascularization in the progression of a tumor, and indicate that vascularization is also an important step in setting the stage for metastatic spread of cancer cells. (Consumer Summary produced by Reliance Medical Information. Inc.) Histologic and clinical characteristics of 49 patients. (table) Metastatic disease among 49 patients. (graph)

BC0808 BREAST CANCER

Weinhouse, B.
Ladies' Home Journal
Aug. 1986, vol. 103, p. 60(1)

BC0809 MARKER PREDICTS BREAST CANCER RECURRENCE

Weiss, R.
Science News
Sept. 9, 1989, vol. 136, n. n11, p. 164(1)
Carrier proteins

BC0810 GENETIC PROPENSITY TO COMMON CANCERS FOUND

Weiss, R.
Science News
Dec. 1, 1990, vol. 138, n. n22, p. 342(1)
Genetic disorders

BC0811 THE MEDICAL MANAGEMENT OF BREAST CANCER

Williams, C.J.
1987, vol. VIII, p. 246

BC0812 GOING BY NUMBERS

Wright, K.
New York Times Magazine
Dec. 15, 1991, p. 58-60, 77, 70
Epidemiology; preventive medicine; cancer research

BC0813 BETTER TREATMENT FOR BREAST CANCER

Young, S.
Glamour
Aug. 1992, vol. 90, n. n8, p. 35(1)

AUTHOR INDEX

SUBJECT INDEX